Acclaim for *It Starts with the Egg*

"Rebecca Fett's stellar constellation of perspective, experience, knowledge, and scientific background may well revolutionize our current global conversation, understanding and practices related to fertility... It is hard to overestimate the impact that this book may have on the lives of many."

- DR. CLAUDIA WELCH, AUTHOR OF *BALANCE YOUR HORMONES, BALANCE YOUR LIFE: ACHIEVING OPTIMAL HEALTH AND WELLNESS THROUGH AYURVEDA, CHINESE MEDICINE, AND WESTERN SCIENCE.*

"With detailed, up to date research Rebecca Fett provides a clear, cool-headed guide to both the science that determines IVF success, and the practical changes that patients can make to drastically increase their chances of IVF success."

- DR. LINDSAY WU, LABORATORY FOR AGEING RESEARCH, UNIVERSITY OF NEW SOUTH WALES MEDICAL CENTER, AUSTRALIA.

"This is a very useful resource: well-researched, accessibly written and with easy-to-follow take-home messages and action plans. I would recommend this to any woman who is trying to conceive."

- DR. CLAIRE DEAKIN, FACULTY OF POPULATION HEALTH SCIENCES, UNIVERSITY COLLEGE LONDON.

"A thoroughly-researched and eye-opening account of how small, simple lifestyle changes can have powerful, positive effects on your health and fertility. A must-read for women wanting the best chance of conceiving a healthy baby."

- BETH GREER, BESTSELLING AUTHOR OF *SUPER NATURAL HOME.*

"It Starts with the Egg presents a reasoned and balanced review of the latest science linking environmental chemicals to reduced fertility and other health problems. Readers will find sound advice for how to avoid chemicals of concern, providing a useful guide for couples that want to improve their chances of a healthy pregnancy."

- DR. LAURA VANDENBERG, UNIVERSITY OF MASSACHUSETTS, AMHERST, SCHOOL OF PUBLIC HEALTH.

"This timely synthesis of scientific literature is essential reading for both women and men wanting practical, evidence-based recommendations to enhance their fertility."

- DR. LORETTA MCKINNON, EPIDEMIOLOGIST, PRINCESS ALEXANDRA HOSPITAL.

"With 'It Starts with the Egg,' Rebecca Fett delivers a much needed overview on the available scientific evidence regarding the influence of nutrition on fertility and fertility treatment, providing a valuable resource for couples trying to conceive."

- DR. JOHN TWIGT, DEPARTMENT OF OBSTETRICS AND GYNECOLOGY, ERASMUS MEDICAL CENTER, NETHERLANDS

"Rebecca has done a great service for all women, children, and future generations by starting at the beginning of a human life and examining which toxic chemicals cause harm to the egg... This book is a wonderful addition to the growing library of information on toxic exposures."

- DEBRA LYNN DADD, AUTHOR OF TOXIC FREE: HOW TO PROTECT YOUR HEALTH AND HOME FROM THE CHEMICALS THAT ARE MAKING YOU SICK

"Rebecca Fett's 'It Starts with the Egg' is a complete guide to everything a woman can do to improve her egg quality before trying to conceive..."It Starts with the Egg" also breaks information down in easy-to-digest bullet points that show exactly what to do to get to where you want to be: the parent of a happy, healthy, gorgeous baby."

- CHERYL ALKON, AUTHOR OF BALANCING PREGNANCY WITH PRE-EXISTING DIABETES: HEALTHY MOM, HEALTHY BABY.

How the **Science of Egg Quality** Can Help You
Get Pregnant Naturally, Prevent Miscarriage,
and **Improve Your Odds in IVF**

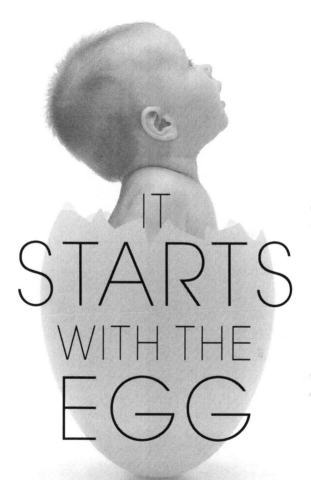

IT
STARTS
WITH THE
EGG

REBECCA FETT

Franklin Fox Publishing
New York

FRANKLIN FOX PUBLISHING
Copyright © 2014, 2016 by Rebecca Fett
Published in the United States by Franklin Fox Publishing LLC,
New York.

Copyeditor: Kira Freed
Interior/Cover Design: Steven Plummer / SPDesign
Front Cover Photo: ©iStock.com/Tsekhmister
Back Cover Photo: Tessa Falk

Library of Congress Control Number: 2014904327

ISBN-13: 978-0991126903
ISBN-10: 0991126904

www.franklinfox.com

Table of Contents

Introduction

"Only I can change my life. No one can do it for me."
— CAROL BURNETT

WHETHER YOU ARE just starting to think about having a baby, find yourself on the long road of fertility treatments and failed IVF cycles, or have suffered multiple miscarriages, it is critically important to provide your eggs with the specific nutrients needed to support embryo development and to avoid the toxins that cause the most harm. This book will explain the simple things you can do to have the best possible chance of getting pregnant and bringing home a healthy baby. And it starts with the egg.

The conventional thinking is that women are born with all the eggs they will ever have and that the quality of those eggs declines drastically with age. But this is not the whole story. Most of our lives, our eggs are in a state of suspended animation as immature cells, but in the three to four months before ovulation, an egg must undergo a major transformation. It grows dramatically in size and starts producing much more energy. The egg must then execute a precise process of separating and ejecting copies of chromosomes. If this process goes wrong, and it often does, the egg will have chromosomal abnormalities. These chromosomal abnormalities are the single most important cause of early miscarriages and failed IVF cycles as well as the reason it takes older women so much longer to conceive.

Many women are told there is little they can do to improve egg quality, but the latest research defies that old assumption. The growth phase before ovulation is a critical time during which many things can happen that affect the quality of the egg, both positively and negatively. These include harmful effects from exposure to toxins such as BPA and phthalates as well as protective effects from added antioxidants and other nutrients. As a result, there is a brief window of opportunity in which you can make a difference to your egg quality.

This book will be your guide to specific strategies that are supported by strong scientific research. Importantly, the advice in this book is not based on isolated animal studies that provide enticing hints as to the causes and solutions for poor egg quality. Individual studies, and particularly animal or test-tube studies, provide only limited evidence and must be taken with a grain of salt. Instead, this book is based on a comprehensive analysis of a large body of medical research involving studies that have been confirmed by multiple groups and that involve real patients.

If you are currently being treated by a fertility specialist, you may have already received advice about supplements that can improve egg quality. The advice of some doctors will be more up-to-date and supported by scientific research than that of others. My goal in writing this book is to provide a tool for thoroughly understanding what helps and why, so you can make your own informed decisions.

But first, the story of how I became obsessed with the science of egg quality. My mission started with the same fears and anxieties faced by many women struggling with infertility. I was about to begin an IVF cycle and could not help worrying, Is this going to work? Will we get enough eggs? Will they produce any embryos that are good enough to transfer and lead to a pregnancy?

In any IVF cycle, there are so many opportunities for things to go wrong and so much at stake. In our IVF cycle, there was also another person counting on me to produce enough eggs: our gestational carrier (or "surrogate"). If this cycle failed, not only would I have to repeat all the injections and doctors' appointments, but so would she.

I had started the process with so much confidence, thinking that since I was under 30, conceiving through IVF would be easy. But then the unexpected happened. I was diagnosed with diminished ovarian reserve and told by our fertility specialist that the most aggressive drug protocol would be required to help us conceive. If they were able to retrieve only a few eggs, our chance of having an embryo to transfer was not good. I asked our fertility specialist if there were any particular supplements I should take that could improve our chances, but there were no clear answers. So I put my training in molecular biology and biochemistry to work. I embarked on a mission to find out for myself what the scientific research showed.

In the process of earning my molecular biology degree, I had studied mechanisms of DNA damage and repair, the detailed process of energy production inside cells, and how both processes relate to antioxidants. I had also studied the complex system in which chromosomes in an egg are recombined and then mechanically separated before and after fertilization. As I delved deeper into the scientific papers addressing egg quality, all the pieces that I had learned about years earlier started to fit together with groundbreaking recent studies to form a picture of the various causes of chromosomal abnormalities in eggs and the influence of external factors. In short, the research revealed a quiet revolution in the way we think about egg quality.

I started putting into practice everything I had learned. I improved my diet by cutting out refined carbohydrates (to lower insulin, which is shown to impact egg quality), started taking a small handful of daily supplements, and took extra steps to limit my exposure to household toxins, such as replacing plastic with glass and buying all-natural cleaning products.

I also decided to take the hormone DHEA, which, as I will explain later in this book, has been the subject of heated debate in the IVF world in the past five years. During those months, I started thinking of myself as "pre-pregnant" and protected my eggs the way I would protect a growing baby if I were pregnant. I found it reassuring that even if this particular IVF cycle failed, I could at least take comfort in the knowledge that I had done absolutely everything I could to make healthy embryos.

That said, I was not expecting any miracles. I still suspected that with a diminished reserve of eggs, I had an uphill battle.

I had seen the statistics showing IVF success rates in relation to ovarian reserve, and they were not grounds for optimism.

A couple of months after beginning my quest for egg quality, my husband and I went back to the fertility clinic for a routine check of my ovaries before starting the IVF stimulation medication. We were shocked to witness how much had changed. Instead of a couple of follicles (the small structures in which a single egg matures) in each ovary, the ultrasound showed that I probably had about 20 eggs maturing. This number was perfectly normal, and I felt the weight of the words "diminished ovarian reserve" lifting from my shoulders. Our odds had suddenly become a lot better.

Nevertheless, I remained nervous. The weeks passed, and each day became a routine of injections, pills, ultrasounds, and blood tests. The tests gave us every reason to expect a good outcome, but as our doctor explained, there are never any guarantees in an IVF cycle because so much can go wrong. Every morning and evening when I took out my boxes of syringes, needles, and vials of expensive fertility drugs, preparing to give myself several injections, I felt a twinge of anxiety, knowing this could all be for nothing.

On the day of the egg retrieval, I woke up after the procedure to discover that they had retrieved 22 eggs, and all were mature. Even through the haze of the anesthetic, this news brought huge relief. I tried not to get too excited, knowing there were still quite a few hurdles to go, but suddenly we were faced with the very real prospect that this cycle could actually work.

At this point, I knew it was a numbers game. In a typical IVF cycle where 20 eggs are retrieved, approximately 15 will fertilize. Of those embryos, only a third are likely to make it to 5-day-old embryos ready to be transferred into the uterus. We planned to do a single embryo transfer, so we needed just one good-quality embryo that made it to this critical 5-day-old "blastocyst" stage. But knowing that a huge proportion of embryo transfers fail and that we might need to do a second or third round of embryo transfer to become pregnant, the more embryos we could get, the better.

Later that day as we waited to find out how many eggs had fertilized, the clinic called. Out of 22 eggs, 19 had fertilized. There was now a very good chance that a few embryos would make it to the blastocyst stage, although many couples in the same position are not so lucky. Five days later, we were in for another surprise. Every single one of our embryos had survived to become a good-quality blastocyst. This result was simply unheard of. In fact, even though our clinic had treated thousands of patients and had one of the highest success rates in the United States, we had easily set a new clinic record for the number of good-quality blastocysts from a single cycle.

On the sixth day after the egg retrieval, we transferred one perfect-looking embryo and began the notoriously difficult two-week wait to find out if our surrogate was pregnant. What happened next was what we all wish for: a positive pregnancy test. It is impossible to know if the same result would have happened without my mission to improve my egg quality, but the scientific research shows that egg quality is the single most important factor in determining whether an egg will fertilize and survive to the blastocyst stage. It also determines whether an embryo is capable of implanting and leading to a viable pregnancy.

As I told this story to my female friends, the reaction was the same regardless of the life stage they were in. Everyone wanted to know what they could do to improve their own chances. I found myself wanting to delve into the scientific research again. It is one thing to make a determination for myself on whether the research shows that a particular supplement is safe and worthwhile, but if I was going to share my knowledge with other women who were trying to get pregnant or who had suffered multiple miscarriages, I had a much greater responsibility to get it right. And so I began an even more exhaustive search and analysis of the latest research relating to egg quality.

I carefully analyzed hundreds of scientific papers investigating specific effects of toxins and nutrients on biological processes, identifying influences on fertility and miscarriage rates in large, population-based studies, and uncovering the factors that influence success rates in IVF. (You can find these scientific papers listed in the references section, along with information on how to access them online.) This comprehensive research was an undertaking most fertility specialists are simply too busy to do, and, unsurprisingly, many doctors are not up-to-date on recent findings.

I quickly learned that the standard advice of IVF clinics and fertility books is simply not keeping pace with research. As just one example, you would be hard-pressed to find a doctor who is knowledgeable about the latest research showing that BPA, a toxin commonly found in plastic food-storage containers, has a significant negative effect on fertility and IVF success rates.

Part of the problem is that much of the research is so recent, such as the studies published in 2012 by researchers at the Harvard School of Public Health that found that women with higher BPA levels in their bloodstream produced fewer eggs and embryos in an IVF cycle, and their embryos were less likely to implant and lead to a pregnancy.[1] The large body of research on BPA provides a powerful reason to do what you can to limit your exposure — but you are unlikely to find out about BPA from your doctor.

This is not to suggest that all IVF clinics are behind the times when it comes to research on supplements and egg quality. Some do stay abreast of the research and recommend a cocktail of supplements that closely aligns with the advice in this book (at time of writing, Colorado Center for Reproductive Medicine [CCRM], for example). But these clinics generally do not explain the fascinating story of how each supplement is thought to work and cannot reach patients outside the IVF context. They also fail to mention all the important measures you can take other than supplements.

Many women preparing for IVF are aware that they may not be getting the most up-to-date advice about what supplements can improve their chances, and so turn to the Internet for information. This path often leads to supplements that are not supported by any scientific research or that may actually be harmful for fertility, such as royal jelly and L-arginine. This book not only discusses the measures that may help but also debunks myths about some supplements that may do more harm than good.

For women trying to conceive naturally instead of through IVF, relying on Internet research to figure out which supplements to take can be particularly problematic because egg quality is not the only issue to consider.

As just one example, research has clearly demonstrated that melatonin supplements improve egg quality and are thus often recommended for women undergoing IVF. But the problem is that taking melatonin supplements long term could potentially disrupt ovulation. This means that melatonin is only helpful in the IVF context, where natural regulation of ovulation is less important. If you are trying to conceive naturally, disrupted ovulation is a significant problem, and taking melatonin could actually make it more difficult to get pregnant. Trawling the Internet for ideas on what to take for fertility is likely to miss these nuances and cause trouble for many women.

The supplement DHEA provides another example of some of the problems with the standard advice of many IVF clinics. If you have been diagnosed with diminished ovarian reserve and are preparing for IVF, whether or not you will be advised to take DHEA depends more on which IVF clinic you happen to be attending rather than any logical basis. Many clinics also leave the decision of whether to take DHEA up to the individual patient, without providing any detailed information about the strength of the clinical evidence. We deserve better and have a right to make truly informed decisions.

Seeing the immense gap between the research and conventional fertility advice, I felt compelled to help by distilling the clinical research into concrete, comprehensible information. As I became more convinced of the impact of external factors on egg quality and how important egg quality is to the chance of conceiving, whether naturally or through IVF, I felt an urgent need to help educate other women struggling with infertility. And so this book was born.

Seeing our growing baby on the 12-week ultrasound and hearing the heart beat were moments of such pure joy that I wanted the same for everyone else going through the process of fertility treatment or planning to have a baby. Of course, in the world of infertility there are never any promises. No one can offer a guaranteed way to get pregnant because there are so many variables and unique challenges, particularly if you are trying to conceive after the age of 35. But this book offers a plan to improve your odds and, in doing so, improve your overall health and prepare your body for a healthy pregnancy.

How to Use This Book

If You Are Just Starting Out

If you have just begun trying to get pregnant and have no reason to expect fertility challenges, you will likely not need to adopt every suggestion in this book to become pregnant. By focusing on the recommendations in the *basic plan* (summarized at the end of the book) and making simple changes, you may be able to get pregnant faster and reduce the risk of miscarriage. This is because even young, healthy women have a significant proportion of abnormal eggs. If the eggs you happen to ovulate for a few months in a row are affected, this will increase the time it takes you to conceive and put you at risk of losing a pregnancy. The recommendations in this book are also beneficial for your overall health and the health of your future baby, particularly the chapters on avoiding specific toxins that have been shown to harm fetal development.

If You Are Having Difficulty Conceiving

If you have been trying to conceive for more than 12 months, or for more than 6 months and you are over the age of 35, it is a good idea to see a fertility specialist to find out whether there is a specific medical cause of infertility that can be addressed. For many, consulting a fertility specialist will uncover physical barriers to getting pregnant, such as scar tissue or blocked fallopian tubes, or will reveal hormonal problems affecting ovulation or implantation.

A specific treatment may be available, or your doctor may recommend IVF to sidestep the underlying cause of your infertility. Either way, it remains important to take steps to improve your egg quality in concert with other specific treatments because egg quality can impact your chance of success, even if it is not the primary cause of your infertility.

If you fall into this category, with a specifically diagnosed physical or hormonal fertility challenge, you should follow the advice in the *intermediate plan*, which includes additional measures that will have further benefit for egg quality and that address ovulation problems. The plan will be slightly modified if you have been diagnosed with polycystic ovary syndrome (PCOS).

PCOS is the most common ovulatory infertility condition. It has a side effect of reducing egg quality in a specific way. If you have PCOS, it is important to adopt the advice in the *intermediate plan* in addition to the specific dietary and supplement recommendations that will counteract the negative impact of PCOS on egg quality. Specific supplements such as myo-inositol have been found to have a significant benefit for women with PCOS because they rebalance hormones and blood sugar, addressing the cause of poor egg quality and restoring ovulation.

If, however, you have received the catch-all diagnosis of "unexplained infertility" or "age-related infertility," you have the most work to do to improve your egg quality, and the most to gain. I recommend following the *advanced plan*, which incorporates additional supplements and other measures that have been studied in women who have had numerous failed IVF cycles. Because it takes about three months for an egg to mature, it is important to start this plan as soon as possible.

Typically, women diagnosed with "unexplained infertility" or "age-related infertility" are advised by fertility clinics to pursue an escalating program of assisted reproduction techniques, starting with medications, then progressing to intrauterine insemination (IUI) and, ultimately, to IVF. These techniques often succeed, but they do so by circumventing, rather than addressing, the real problem, and there are often many failed attempts along the way.

As the next chapter explains, the rapid decline in fertility that begins in the mid-30s is largely a product of declining egg quality, and this often becomes a limiting factor to becoming pregnant, even with the assistance of IVF. The success rates in IVF cycles are very much dependent on age.[2] Unless donor eggs are used, IVF can only do so much.

If your infertility is either unexplained or has been put down to age, or you have had failed IVF cycles, improving your egg quality should be your primary focus in trying to conceive. Research shows that only good-quality eggs are likely to become good-quality embryos that can survive the critical first week and successfully implant to result in a pregnancy. Whether you choose to pursue IVF or continue trying to conceive naturally, it is critical that you maximize the proportion of eggs that are of good quality and have the potential to become a healthy baby.

Recurrent Miscarriage

Improving egg quality could also play an important role in preventing some types of miscarriages. If you have had more than one miscarriage, your doctor probably recommended a full screening to determine the possible cause. If you have not yet had this screening done, you should insist on it. Many women who have lost multiple pregnancies have blood-clotting or immune disorders that can be treated with medication. Another common cause is an underactive thyroid gland.[3] By finding out if you have one of these medical causes of miscarriage, which explain about a quarter of miscarriages, you may be able to reduce the chance of it happening again. For example, in women who have antibodies attacking their thyroid (known as Hashimoto's thyroiditis), treatment with an added thyroid hormone called levothyroxin reduces the miscarriage rate by more than 50%.[4]

If testing rules out clotting, immune, or thyroid problems as the cause of your pregnancy losses, the most likely culprit is egg quality. This is because a poor-quality egg with chromosomal abnormalities will develop into an embryo and then fetus with chromosomal abnormalities and very little chance of surviving. Chromosomal abnormalities are in fact the most common cause of early miscarriage, accounting for 40–50% of miscarriages.[5]

As the next chapter explains, these chromosomal abnormalities almost always originate in the egg and become even more frequent with age.[6] In this book, you will learn how chromosomal abnormalities often occur during the last phase of egg maturation before ovulation and what you can do to reduce the chance of your next pregnancy being affected.

If you have had two or more miscarriages and your doctor cannot find a medical cause, or you know that chromosomal abnormalities affected your previous pregnancies (such as Down syndrome or another "trisomy"), you may want to consider following the *advanced plan* for at least three months before trying to conceive again.

What About the Sperm?

While the focus of this book is egg quality, many of the same external factors impact sperm in a similar way, as discussed in Chapter 12. Although often not as critical as egg quality, sperm quality can in some cases have a significant effect on your likelihood of conceiving, and it is time to rethink the assumption that the father's age and lifestyle factors are irrelevant. If you know or suspect that male factor infertility is part of your challenge in conceiving, it will be particularly valuable to apply the recommendations in Chapter 12, which explains the specific nutrients that affect sperm quality. Even if you have no cause for concern about sperm quality, you will learn why it is important for all men trying to conceive to take a daily multivitamin to increase the chance of success.

Conclusion

Whether you are trying to conceive naturally, pursuing IVF, or trying again after a pregnancy loss, it is imperative that you do what you can to improve your egg quality. It takes approximately three months for an immature egg to develop into a mature egg ready for ovulation, and this is the crucial window of time for preserving egg quality. In subsequent chapters, you will learn the most important things you can do, but to understand how these lifestyle factors can improve egg quality, it is necessary to first understand what egg quality means and how chromosomal abnormalities occur. That is the subject of Chapter 1.

Part 1

WHAT YOUR DOCTOR **ISN'T** **TELLING YOU**

CHAPTER 1

Understanding Egg Quality

"When you know better you do better."
— Maya Angelou

THE DECLINE IN fertility as we age is almost entirely a result of the decline in egg quantity and quality. We know this because older women who use donor eggs have pregnancy rates similar to younger women. But what does egg quality mean? Broadly, it describes the potential of an egg to become a viable pregnancy after fertilization. And this is no trivial matter — the vast majority of fertilized eggs simply do not have what it takes.

Egg Quality Is Everything

For any embryo, the first few weeks after fertilization represent a major hurdle, and many embryos stop developing at some point during this time. In fact, most naturally conceived embryos are lost before a woman even knows she is pregnant.[1] Only about a third of fertilized embryos actually survive to become a baby.[2] The odds may be even worse in the IVF context, where many fertilized eggs are unable to progress to the five-day embryo stage (known as the "blastocyst" stage), and those that do make it to this stage and are transferred to the uterus often do not successfully implant, resulting in a failed IVF cycle.

The fact that most fertilized eggs never become a successful pregnancy is an issue that receives very little attention because there is a common misconception that getting an egg fertilized is the real challenge in conceiving. Most natural fertility advice therefore focuses on ovulation and timing to achieve fertilization. This approach misses the mark because the potential of a fertilized egg to continue developing is often a much bigger issue. In reality, egg quality plays a critical role in how long it takes to become pregnant, whether naturally or through IVF, and the secret is in the egg's DNA.

Although an embryo's potential to develop into a pregnancy depends on many factors, by far the most important is having the correct number of copies of each chromosome. Chromosomal abnormalities in eggs have a profound impact on fertility because at every stage of development from fertilization onward, an embryo formed from a chromosomally abnormal egg has much less potential to continue developing.[3] This may manifest as an inability to get pregnant or as early miscarriage. For many women, chromosomal abnormalities in eggs become the greatest obstacle to conceiving and carrying to term.

It comes as no surprise that poor egg quality is significantly more common in women who have had a difficult time conceiving. High rates of chromosomal abnormalities are seen in eggs of women who have a history of multiple miscarriages, women who have had repeated IVF cycles in which embryos were transferred but no pregnancy occurred (so-called "repeated implantation failure"), and women with polycystic ovary syndrome. For example, the proportion of abnormal embryos in women with a history of repeated implantation failures in IVF cycles can be up to 70%.[4]

Chromosomal errors in eggs not only impact the ability to get pregnant but are also a major cause of miscarriage. Miscarriages are unfortunately very common, occurring in about 10–15% of recognized pregnancies.[5] However most pregnancy losses are not even noticed because they happen so early — before the woman knows she is pregnant. When such pregnancies are taken into account, up to 70% end in miscarriage.[6] Part of the reason for this incredibly high rate is that from the moment of conception, a continuous process of selection against chromosomally abnormal embryos is taking place.

In fact, *chromosomal abnormalities cause more miscarriages than every other known cause of miscarriage combined.* In one study in Japan involving almost 500 women with a history of 2 or more miscarriages, 41% of miscarriages were found to be caused by a chromosomal abnormality in the fetus, whereas all the other known causes of miscarriage together accounted for less than 30% of pregnancy losses.[7] Other studies have found that more than half of all first-trimester miscarriages are caused by chromosomal abnormalities.[8] It is also important to note that these studies were investigating miscarriages from recognized pregnancies only, and the rate of chromosomal abnormalities is likely to be much higher for losses that occur in the short time after fertilization.[9]

A common reaction to this information is that chromosomal errors in eggs are beyond our control, but recent scientific research is showing that is not true. The proportion of eggs with chromosomal abnormalities can be influenced by nutrients and lifestyle factors you can control. As will be discussed later in this chapter, research suggests that one way external factors can influence egg quality is by boosting or compromising the egg's potential to produce energy at critical times — energy that provides the fuel for proper chromosome processing.

The best-known example of a chromosomal abnormality originating in the egg is Down syndrome, which becomes much more common as women age and egg quality declines. In 95% of cases, Down syndrome is caused by the egg providing an extra copy of chromosome 21, which results in the fetus having three copies instead of the usual two.[10] For this reason, Down syndrome is also called Trisomy 21.

Down syndrome is just one example of a chromosomal abnormality, but it is perhaps the best known because it is one of the few in which the affected fetus can survive to term. Some babies with Trisomy 13 or Trisomy 18 (an extra copy of chromosome 13 or 18) can also survive to term, but with life-threatening medical problems. An extra copy of other chromosomes will prevent the embryo from developing past the first few days or weeks, or will cause an early miscarriage.[11] This is why we rarely hear about chromosomal errors involving extra copies of these other chromosomes, even though they are very common.

While having an extra copy of a chromosome is the most

common type of chromosomal abnormality, occasionally a missing chromosome or more complex errors can also occur.

An egg with the incorrect number of chromosomes is called "aneuploid." An embryo created from one of these aneuploid eggs will also be aneuploid and will have very little potential to successfully implant in the uterus. Even when aneuploid embryos are able to progress to a pregnancy, the vast majority of such pregnancies end in an early miscarriage.[12]

In women over 40, more than half of eggs may be chromosomally abnormal.[13] In fact, by some measures, the rate of abnormalities in women over 40 is as high as 70–80%.[14] Studying chromosomal abnormalities in eggs, we see an exponential increase in the fertility challenge faced with age, starting in the mid- to late 30s. But egg quality has an impact in all age groups, and chromosomal errors in younger women are much more common than you might expect.

Even in women under 35, up to a quarter of eggs are aneuploid on average.[15] This means that if you are a young, healthy woman without any fertility issues, there will still be many ovulation cycles in which you have little potential to conceive. If the egg that you ovulate in a given month is chromosomally abnormal and unable to support a pregnancy, using ovulation prediction kits and charts to achieve fertilization with perfect timing will not make any difference; you will probably not be able to conceive until the next cycle in which you ovulate a good egg.

The dramatic impact of chromosomal abnormalities on the chance of conceiving and carrying to term is particularly apparent in the IVF context. If this factor is taken out of the equation, the pregnancy rates skyrocket. We know this from an exciting new approach to IVF in which embryos are first screened for abnormalities in every chromosome, and only the normal embryos are transferred.

This is very different from the traditional measure of "embryo quality" in the IVF context, which is based on the growth rate and overall appearance of the embryo. A slow-growing embryo with irregular-looking cells is less likely to lead to a pregnancy, but it has become clear in recent years that assessment of embryo quality based on appearance or "morphology" is no guarantee. What matters much more is screening for embryos that have normal chromosomes.

When comprehensive chromosome screening was introduced for poor-prognosis patients at a leading IVF clinic in 2010, the difference was dramatic. Instead of the usual 13% of transferred embryos successfully implanting for patients 41–42 years old, selecting only chromosomally normal embryos boosted the implantation rate to 38%. As a result, the proportion of women in this age group completing an IVF cycle who actually took home a baby *doubled*.[16]

The technique of comprehensive chromosome screening to identify the best embryos was pioneered at the Colorado Center for Reproductive Medicine (CCRM) by Dr. William Schoolcraft, a highly regarded fertility specialist and the author of several studies showing the success of this approach.

Dr. Schoolcraft's studies include many examples of individual patients who were able to conceive only after chromosomally normal embryos were chosen for transfer.[17] One patient mentioned in Dr. Schoolcraft's 2009 study was a 37-year-old who had gone through 6 previous IVF cycles in which the transferred embryos did not implant. She then began yet another IVF cycle, this time with chromosomal screening on 10 of her embryos. Out of those 10 embryos, 7 were found to be chromosomally abnormal. If screening had not been done and embryos had been chosen for transfer by appearance alone, there would have been a high probability of transferring chromosomally abnormal embryos. Those embryos would most likely have failed to implant or led to a miscarriage. Instead of taking that chance, her doctors transferred the 3 chromosomally normal embryos, and she became pregnant with twins.

Another patient in Dr. Schoolcraft's study was a 33-year-old woman who had suffered six miscarriages. In her next IVF cycle, chromosomal screening revealed that out of 11 embryos, 8 had chromosomal errors. Without screening, there was a good chance that 1 of the 8 abnormal embryos would have been transferred, likely resulting in no pregnancy or a seventh miscarriage. Instead, her doctors were able to select 2 chromosomally normal embryos, and she gave birth to twins.

Sometimes chromosomal screening reveals just how heavily the odds can be stacked against a successful pregnancy. This is apparent in Dr. Schoolcraft's example of a 41-year-old woman who was able to conceive after chromosomal screening identified the single embryo out of 8 that was chromosomally normal and had the potential for a normal, healthy pregnancy.

While chromosomal screening represents a very significant advance, it is not a cure-all. One of the main problems is that screening may show that none of the embryos created in an IVF cycle are chromosomally normal. As a result, there will be no good embryo available to transfer. This happened to about a third of patients in one study,[18] demonstrating that egg quality will still remain a limiting factor to becoming pregnant, even with new screening methods.

Yet chromosomal screening does hold great promise and shows the dramatic impact of egg and embryo quality on pregnancy rates. Interestingly, this impact is not limited to "poor-prognosis patients." A group in Japan set out to determine how much they could improve pregnancy rates in IVF cycles by choosing to transfer only chromosomally normal embryos, but this time they were looking at women under 35 with a good prognosis and no previous miscarriages.[19] In the control group, in which embryos were chosen by appearance alone, 41% of patients became pregnant per IVF cycle and carried to at least 20 weeks. In the group in which embryos were chosen by chromosomal screening, the pregnancy rate jumped to 69%. The miscarriage rates were also very different: 9% in the control group and just 2.6% in the screened group.

The lesson we can take away from the positive results of chromosomal screening is that having a chromosomally normal embryo has a huge impact on the chance of a successful pregnancy, no matter how you are trying to conceive. Even if trying to conceive naturally, your chance of becoming pregnant and carrying to term is very much determined by your egg quality. Luckily, egg quality is not entirely predetermined by your age or fixed in time. It can change.

There is, in fact, an enormous variation in chromosomal abnormality rates between different women of the same age.[20] One 35-year-old may ovulate very few chromosomally normal eggs over a given time frame, while another woman's eggs may all be normal at the same age. This was shown in a study of IVF patients in Germany and Italy in which the percentage of chromosomally normal eggs ranged greatly between different women of the same age. The number of normal eggs also varied widely over time for each woman, which was seen as a significant difference in the proportion of normal eggs between two consecutive IVF cycles. The researchers described the variation over time and between different women as random and unpredictable, but only because they did not connect their research to the many other studies showing specific influences on the rates of chromosomal abnormalities. The fascinating research discussed in the remainder of this book establishes that this variability is not purely random; on the contrary, a wide range of external factors impact egg quality.

Countless clinical studies have shown that avoiding certain toxins and adding specific supplements can increase the percentage of eggs that can develop into a good-quality embryo, increase the percentage of embryos that implant in the uterus, and reduce the risk of early-pregnancy loss. There is strong scientific evidence that some of these improvements are due to a reduction in the proportion of eggs with chromosomal abnormalities, confirming the fact that egg quality is something we have the power to change.

How Do Eggs Become "Chromosomally Abnormal"?

The process of egg production is very long and error-prone. The development of each egg begins before a woman is even born, in the newly forming ovaries during the first trimester of pregnancy. A girl is born with all the eggs she will ever have, and each egg exists in a state of suspended animation until a few months before ovulation.

Approximately four months before ovulation, a small pool of immature eggs begin to grow, and while most will die off naturally, one lead egg is selected from the pool to finish maturing.[21] The fully grown egg completes ovulation by bursting from its follicle and traveling down the fallopian tube, ready to be fertilized.

During the decades-long interval between early egg development and ovulation, eggs have many opportunities to accumulate damage as a part of normal aging. The traditional belief is that by the time a woman is 40, her eggs have already accumulated chromosomal abnormalities, and nothing can be done to change that. But that is not scientifically correct, because most chromosomal errors actually occur shortly before ovulation, in later stages of a process called "meiosis."

An egg ends up with the incorrect number of chromosomes when meiosis goes awry. Meiosis involves carefully aligning chromosome copies along the middle of the egg, then pulling one set to each end of the egg with a network of microscopic tubules. One set of chromosomes is then pushed out of the egg in what is called a "polar body." A developing egg actually does this twice — it starts out with four copies of each chromosome and, if the process goes correctly, ends up with just one copy of each chromosome.

If this process fails at any stage, the end result is an extra or missing copy of a chromosome. Although the first round of meiosis begins before a girl is born, most of the chromosomal processing activity happens in the months immediately before an egg is ovulated.

The critical point to note — and a point that many fertility doctors are not aware of — is that most of the chromosomal abnormalities in eggs do not accumulate gradually over 30 or 40 years as an egg ages, but instead happen in the couple of months before an egg is ovulated. In other words, aging does not directly cause chromosomal abnormalities; rather, it creates conditions that predispose eggs to mature incorrectly shortly before ovulation.[22]

This means that by changing those conditions before ovulation, you can increase the odds of an egg maturing with the correct number of chromosomes. In short, you may be able to influence the quality of eggs that you ovulate a couple of months from now because chromosomal errors in those eggs have probably not occurred yet.

This leads us to the fundamental issue: How can an egg be predisposed to mature with an incorrect number of chromosomes, and what can you do about it? Every chapter in this book addresses different aspects of that question, but a common theme is the egg's energy supply.

Energy Production in the Egg

It takes an enormous amount of energy for the egg to process chromosomes correctly and do all the other work necessary to mature properly. It turns out that the energy-producing structures inside eggs change significantly with age and in response to nutrients and other external factors.[23] These structures, called "mitochondria," are found in nearly every cell in the body. They act as miniature power plants to transform various fuel sources into energy that the cell can use, in the form of ATP.

ATP is quite literally the energy of life. It moves muscles, makes enzymes work, and powers nerve impulses. Just about every other biological process depends on it. And it is the primary form of energy used by eggs. A growing egg needs a lot of ATP and has a lot of mitochondria. In fact, each egg has more than fifteen thousand mitochondria — over ten times more than any other cell in the body.[24] The follicle cells surrounding the egg also contain many mitochondria and supply the egg with additional ATP.[25] But these mitochondria must be in good condition to make enough energy.

Over time, and in response to oxidative stress (explained in Chapter 6), mitochondria become damaged and less able to produce energy.[26] Without sufficient energy, egg and embryo development may go awry or stop altogether.[27] As explained by Dr. Robert Casper, a leading fertility specialist in Toronto, "the ageing female reproductive system is like a forgotten flashlight on the top shelf of a closet. When you stumble across it a few years later and try to switch it on, it won't work, not because there's anything wrong with the flashlight but because the batteries inside it have died."[28] A growing body of evidence suggests that the ability of an egg to produce energy when needed is critically important to being able to mature with the correct number of chromosomes. It is also vital to an embryo's potential to survive the first week and successfully implant.

Poorly functioning mitochondria may be one of the most important reasons some women's eggs are more likely to end up with chromosomal abnormalities or otherwise lack the potential to become a viable embryo. What you can do to help "recharge" your mitochondria and thereby boost your eggs' energy supply is the subject of several chapters later in this book, but first we turn to another contributor to chromosomal errors in developing eggs — the toxin BPA.

CHAPTER 2

The Dangers of BPA

*"The most exciting phrase to hear in science,
the one that heralds new discoveries, is not
'Eureka!' (I found it!) but 'That's funny ... '"*

— ISAAC ASIMOV

IF YOU WANT the best possible chance of becoming pregnant and delivering a healthy baby, one of the first steps you should take is to reduce your exposure to specific toxins that can harm fertility. This subject has long been neglected in traditional fertility books and in doctors' offices, but it is incredibly important to learn about if you are trying to conceive.

One toxin that has been proven to compromise egg quality and fertility is BPA, which stands for Bisphenol A. This chemical is still commonly used in everything from plastic food containers to paper receipts, despite years of public attention about its potential health dangers.

This chapter will arm you with the resources you need to minimize your exposure to BPA — illustrating how small, simple changes can have powerful positive effects on your health and fertility.

Where We Are

If any chemical deserves its bad press, it is BPA. Even after intense lobbying to ban BPA because of the risks it poses to the health of babies, children, and adults, one impact of BPA has not received as much attention as it deserves: the risk it poses to fertility. The latest research shows that even minuscule amounts of BPA can interfere with hormonal systems and harm developing eggs, compromising success rates in IVF and increasing miscarriage risk.

While much of the research on BPA and fertility is brand new, it fits together with decades of science showing the general health risks of BPA. In fact, so much is known about the health risks of BPA and so many products now say "BPA-free" that one might be tempted to assume that companies have stopped using this nasty chemical and the danger has passed. Unfortunately, that is not the case, and until there is genuine government regulation, it will remain up to each individual to guard against bringing BPA into the home. But the good news is that you can easily reduce your exposure once you know how.

The Case Against BPA

The story of BPA and fertility begins with a chance discovery so unexpected that researchers spent years verifying their results before going public. Dr. Patricia Hunt and her research group at Case Western Reserve University were using laboratory mice to study egg development and saw something very unusual in

August 1998: a dramatic increase in the number of chromo-somally abnormal eggs. In mice, typically only 1–2% of eggs are unable to properly align the chromosomes in the middle of the egg. However, in Dr. Hunt's laboratory, this specific problem suddenly spiked and affected 40% of the eggs, along with other severe chromosomal aberrations. When the eggs matured, they were much more likely to have an incorrect number of chromo-somes. As Dr. Hunt observed, "I was really horrified because we saw this night and day change."[1]

The researchers began a thorough investigation and eventu-ally found the culprit. BPA had started leaching out of the mice's plastic cages and water bottles after they were washed with deter-gent. When all of these damaged plastic cages and bottles were replaced, the rate of eggs with chromosomal errors began to return to normal. Dr. Hunt's group did not publish this finding for several years, though, because the implications for human fertility were so troubling that the researchers wanted to do fur-ther investigation to make sure they were right.[2] "This chemical that we're all exposed to could be causing an increase in miscar-riages and birth defects." Dr. Hunt recalls thinking, "I'm really worried about that."[3]

To confirm that BPA was the specific cause of the egg abnor-malities, the researchers gave controlled doses of BPA to the mice — and the same thing happened. Through a series of investigations over several years, the group determined that even a low dose of BPA during the final stages of egg development is enough to interfere with meiosis and cause chromosomal abnor-malities in eggs. The researchers commented that their findings had obvious relevance for chromosomal errors in human eggs because of the extraordinary similarity in chromosome processing between the two species.[4]

After Dr. Hunt's discovery, other researchers continued to study how BPA could affect fertility and soon uncovered further evidence that BPA is not only toxic to developing eggs but also interferes with the hormones that carefully coordinate the reproductive system.

In the past 15 years, study after study has shown that the small amount of BPA we are all exposed to on a daily basis could have serious health implications. The suspected toxic effects are wide-ranging and include diabetes, obesity, heart disease, and impacts on the brain and reproductive system of infants exposed during pregnancy.[5] Dr. Hunt remarked that "all of the work we've done on BPA only really increases my concern."

In 2008, one of the first large-scale studies was published showing the effects of BPA exposure on human health. Dr. Iain Lang and his colleagues analyzed data collected by the Centers for Disease Control (CDC) from over 1,000 people and found a link between BPA exposure and diabetes, heart disease, and liver toxicity.[6]

These findings, which were subsequently confirmed by other large-scale studies,[7] were cause for concern because BPA is so widely used. Although some companies then worked to remove BPA from their products, it remains very common. Some of the worst offenders are products many people use on a daily basis: plastic food storage containers, canned food and drinks, and paper receipts.

BPA most often enters the body when people consume food

and drinks that have been packaged or stored in a material that leaches BPA, but small amounts can also be absorbed through the skin from contact with products coated with BPA, such as paper receipts. By either path, BPA makes its way into the bloodstream and then into various tissues. As a result, measurable levels can be found in more than 95% of the U.S. population.[8] Over 20 peer-reviewed publications have also reported measurable BPA in the bloodstream in a range of populations all over the world.[9]

Hundreds of studies have now shown that BPA has toxic effects in animals at the same levels that people are exposed to on a daily basis. While BPA causes a vast array of different biological effects once in the bloodstream, perhaps the most troubling effects involve hormonal systems. BPA has consistently been found to interfere with the activity of estrogen, testosterone, and thyroid hormones.[10] Because of this interference with endocrine systems, BPA is called an "endocrine disruptor."

It is not altogether surprising that BPA interferes with hormonal systems, because it has long been known to mimic estrogen. It was originally identified as a synthetic form of estrogen in 1936, when pharmaceutical companies were searching for a drug they could use in hormone treatment. But stronger chemicals were identified a short time later, so BPA was quickly abandoned for those purposes. Yet BPA is actually not as weak as first thought.

BPA used to be considered a "weak estrogen" because it binds to the traditional estrogen receptor about 10,000 times less strongly than estrogen does.[11] However, we now know that estrogen works through a number of different receptors and pathways. And BPA in fact binds to some of these other receptors and has biological effects with the same potency as estrogen.[12] As a result of those findings, BPA can no longer be called a "weak" endocrine disruptor. Hormonal systems are so finely tuned to regulate biological functions throughout the body that even a tiny dose of a chemical such as BPA can cause big problems.

Are Companies Really Still Allowed to Use BPA?

In response to the large body of research on the dangers of BPA, there has been strong public pressure for regulatory agencies to take action and ban BPA. But in most jurisdictions, very little has been done. Those governments that have banned BPA have typically limited the ban to items such as baby bottles. This is a good first step because infants are likely to be particularly vulnerable to BPA, but it does not go far enough.

As Dr. Hunt exclaimed, "what the heck is this stuff doing in consumer products, and especially products that are containers for food and beverages, if we know it's a synthetic estrogen? That really makes me mad."

In 2011, the FDA banned BPA from baby bottles and sippy cups, but in the words of the Environmental Working Group, this move was "purely cosmetic." Manufacturers had already switched to BPA-free plastic in baby bottles in response to consumer demand, and the FDA's decision was prompted by a request from a chemical industry trade association, which believed that a ban would boost consumer confidence in plastic products.[13]

In response, the Environmental Working Group observed that "if the agency truly wants to prevent people from being exposed to this toxic chemical associated with a variety of serious and chronic conditions it should ban its use in cans of infant formula, food and beverages." The Natural Resources Defense Council also described the move as halfhearted and inadequate, criticizing the FDA for dodging the bigger question of BPA's safety.[14]

Even after prohibiting the use of BPA in baby bottles, the FDA maintained that BPA is safe. In March 2012, the FDA concluded that "the scientific evidence at this time does not suggest that the very low levels of human exposure to BPA through the diet are unsafe."[15] It is difficult to understand how the FDA could espouse this position in the face of hundreds of studies showing that BPA is harmful, but it appears that the FDA may have overlooked sound research showing BPA's toxicity in favor of research funded by the plastics industry.

In 2008, the FDA issued a "draft assessment" on the safety of BPA, stating that exposure levels to BPA from food contact materials are below those that may cause health effects.[16] In reaching this conclusion, the FDA relied primarily on two animal studies showing that BPA has no effect[17] but disregarded approximately one hundred studies by government-funded researchers showing that BPA has a range of health effects even at the low doses people are exposed to on a daily basis.[18]

The studies that the FDA relied on were funded by Polycarbonate/BPA Global Group, which represents the manufacturers of BPA and plastics containing BPA.[19] As experts quickly observed, these industry-funded studies were seriously flawed.[20] Among many other shortcomings, the studies used a strain of mice known to have very low sensitivity to hormones and therefore predicted to be much less sensitive to BPA than humans.[21]

Even the peer review panel assembled by the FDA to review its findings criticized the FDA's selection of research publications to rely on. This panel of experts from academic research institutions and the CDC stated that it disagreed "with the decision by FDA to dismiss many other studies on BPA that…were otherwise scientifically sound, inclusive of more advanced and sensitive endpoints, and that were often indicative of BPA impacts that could potentially portend significant risks to health at lower levels of exposure…."[22]

In other words, it appears that the FDA concluded that BPA poses no harm by ignoring high-quality research that investigated subtler effects of BPA at low doses. And the FDA ignored these studies in favor of research funded by the plastics industry.

The clear consensus among academic researchers is that BPA poses a range of health dangers. We should not be reassured by the official government positions that BPA is not harmful. It often takes an incredibly long time for governments to acknowledge that chemicals are unsafe and to prohibit their use, as evidenced by the decades-long battles over lead, PCBs, and asbestos, even in the face of clear evidence of harm.

Instead of waiting for government action, you can choose for yourself whether you want to err on the side of caution and take steps to avoid exposure to BPA. Doing so is particularly important if you are trying to conceive because there is strong scientific evidence that BPA is a threat to fertility and is toxic to developing babies during pregnancy.

How BPA Affects Fertility

A couple of years after Dr. Hunt's accidental experiment showing the effect of BPA on eggs from laboratory mice, evidence began to emerge that BPA significantly impairs fertility in humans too. We now know that women with high levels of BPA in their system during an IVF cycle end up with fewer embryos to transfer and are less likely to become pregnant.

One of the first studies hinting at this, published in 2008, showed a worrisome correlation: higher BPA levels in women who did not achieve pregnancy in IVF compared with those who did.[23] This study was troubling, but it was not until 2011 and 2012 that a body of research was published firmly establishing that anyone facing infertility should be thinking about how to limit exposure to BPA.

In 2011, a group of leading researchers and fertility specialists evaluated the link between BPA and IVF outcomes in 58 women undergoing an IVF cycle at the University of California, San Francisco Center for Reproductive Health. They found that eggs retrieved from women with higher BPA levels were less likely to fertilize.[24] This finding strongly suggests that BPA exposure reduces egg quality, which has implications not just for IVF patients but for all women trying to conceive.

These harmful effects of BPA start even before the fertilization stage. Another study the same year found that BPA impacts the ovarian response to IVF stimulation medication. In that study, women with higher BPA levels had fewer eggs retrieved and lower estrogen levels.[25] On a practical level, this research indicates that BPA appears to disrupt egg development and that if you have had an IVF cycle fail due to a low egg number, BPA could be one of the contributing factors.

The discovery that BPA could compromise IVF cycles was confirmed in 2012 by researchers at the Harvard School of Public Health. In a comprehensive study of 174 women undergoing IVF at the Massachusetts General Hospital Fertility Center in Boston, the researchers found that women with higher BPA levels had fewer eggs retrieved, lower estrogen levels, and a lower fertilization rate.[26] The women with above-average BPA levels also had fewer five-day old embryos available to transfer. For some women, this decrease in embryo number could mean the difference between getting pregnant and having to start the IVF process all over again.

The same Harvard researchers also found that the impact of BPA does not end with the number of eggs and embryos formed. They also showed a link between BPA concentration in women and the failure of embryos to implant and lead to a pregnancy.[27]

The concept of implantation failure was discussed in detail in Chapter 1. To review briefly, in both natural conception and IVF, only a minority of embryos are able to implant in the uterus and develop into a viable pregnancy. Implantation failure is one of the major causes of unsuccessful IVF cycles.

The Harvard researchers found that the odds of implantation failure increased with increasing levels of urinary BPA. The difference in implantation rate between women with high and low BPA levels was dramatic: The quarter of women with the highest BPA exposure had almost twice the odds of implantation failure compared to the quarter of women with the lowest BPA levels.

The researchers also observed that BPA had a bigger impact on the rate of implantation in certain groups of women. Specifically, women with diminished ovarian reserve (which becomes common with age) seemed to be more sensitive to the effects of BPA.

The Harvard researchers speculated that BPA not only decreases egg quality but may also interfere with the environment of the uterus in a way that reduces the ability of embryos to implant. This decrease in "uterine receptivity" had previously been observed in animals exposed to BPA but is not yet fully understood in humans.[28] One of the ways BPA is now thought to interfere with implantation is by interfering with hormone signaling in the cells that line the uterus.

In addition, there is some limited evidence that BPA may impact miscarriage rates. In a small study in Japan, 45 women with a history of 3 or more first-trimester miscarriages had their BPA levels measured and compared to the BPA levels of 32 healthy women with no history of fertility problems. The researchers found that the average BPA level in the women with recurrent miscarriage was about *three times* higher than in the control group.[29]

In another recent study, BPA was again implicated in raising the risk of miscarriage.[30] Researchers from Stanford University, the University of Missouri, and the University of California, San Francisco tested BPA levels in 114 women who had recently become pregnant and who all had trouble getting pregnant or had a history of miscarriage. The researchers divided the women into 4 groups according to their BPA levels and were able to cor-relate the amount of BPA in their blood serum with their risk of miscarrying. Women in the top quartile of BPA had an 80% greater risk of miscarriage than women in the lowest quartile.

Beyond initial studies, very little is known about the impact of BPA on miscarriage rates. But an increased miscarriage risk fits with the research showing that BPA impacts fertilization and implantation rates in women undergoing IVF because we know that at the root of all three outcomes is egg quality. Specifically, only an egg with normal chromosomes has a good chance of fertilizing, implanting, and leading to an ongoing pregnancy, whereas an egg with chromosomal abnormalities is less likely to make it at each stage and more likely to lead to a miscarriage.

If BPA causes chromosomal abnormalities in eggs, we would expect to see lower rates of fertilization, embryo survival, and implantation, and a higher risk of early miscarriage, which is exactly what has been observed. There is also very strong direct evidence that BPA exposure during the critical window of egg development does in fact cause chromosomal abnormalities.

In the years following Dr. Hunt's accidental discovery that BPA causes chromosomal abnormalities in the eggs of mice, further research in animals has begun to uncover exactly how and when this happens.

In 2008, Dr. Sandy Lenie found that a low dose of BPA given continuously as eggs matured caused twice as many chromosomally abnormal eggs compared to eggs that had not been exposed to BPA. These abnormalities were mainly due to failure of chromosomes to align properly; the chromosomes were scattered throughout the egg instead of being arranged in an orderly way so that the cell could divide them properly.

Another study discovered that the later part of egg development is particularly sensitive to BPA; it was found that a high level of BPA exposure shortly before ovulation was enough to halt development of some eggs and cause severe chromosomal abnormalities in any eggs that did mature.[31]

Scientists are now beginning to understand how BPA causes these problems in developing eggs. It appears that BPA interferes with the scaffold-like structures of tubules that organize and separate chromosomes during egg development.[32] These tubules play such a critical role in the process of meiosis that if they cannot work properly, egg development will stop altogether or will go awry, resulting in severe chromosomal abnormalities. Numerous studies suggest that this is at least one way in which BPA is toxic to eggs.[33]

The fact that BPA interferes with egg development can explain much of what is seen in IVF cycles, but there is likely much more to the story because the effects of BPA are even more widespread.

It has been firmly established that BPA also disrupts the hormone systems that are vitally important for fertility. Hormones are signaling molecules that tell the body what to do and when. The activity of the reproductive system is carefully orchestrated by the precise concentration of different hormones and changes in hormone levels over time.

Perhaps one of the most important hormones in female fertility is estrogen. It has many jobs to do in the ovaries, uterus, brain, and other parts of the body. For example, estrogen stimulates ovarian follicles to grow. This is important because each developing ovarian follicle contains an egg, and as a follicle grows and matures, so does the egg within. Without sufficient levels of hormones such as estrogen that stimulate the follicle to grow further, the egg may not continue maturing.

BPA decreases the production of estrogen in the ovaries. In 2013, it was discovered that BPA likely does this by disrupting production of the proteins that help make estrogen.[34] Many other studies have also shown that BPA alters hormone production in the cells of ovarian follicles.[35] BPA also appears to impact fertility by blocking the ability of estrogen to bind to its receptors.[36] In short, BPA interferes with a very precisely controlled hormonal system in a variety of ways.

Estrogen is not the only target of BPA, however. BPA also disrupts other hormonal systems, such as testosterone, thyroid hormones, and insulin, all of which are relevant to egg development and fertility.[37] Given this disruption of critical fertility hormones, it is not at all surprising that BPA impairs ovarian follicle growth and increases the rate at which the ovarian follicles die off.[38]

BPA and PCOS

Limiting your exposure to BPA could be especially helpful if you are one of the millions of women with diabetes, polycystic ovary syndrome (PCOS), or both. PCOS is a very common syndrome that results in ovulation problems and a much harder time conceiving. A hallmark of PCOS is that the body does not respond to insulin as it should. The muscles and tissues become less sensitive to insulin's message to take up sugar from the bloodstream, resulting in higher blood sugar levels and higher insulin levels. This state, which is called "insulin resistance," is also characteristic of diabetes.

Women with diabetes and/or PCOS often have lower egg quality and difficulty getting pregnant.[39] Later chapters will describe the specific dietary strategies and supplements that are helpful to improving egg quality in the context of PCOS and diabetes, but there is also good evidence pointing to BPA as a contributing factor to these conditions.

Several studies have found that BPA levels are significantly higher in women with PCOS.[40] BPA levels are also strongly associated with the hormonal and metabolic changes characteristic of PCOS, and women with higher BPA levels tend to have greater insulin resistance and higher levels of insulin and testosterone.

Large studies have also shown a strong link between BPA levels and diabetes.[41] For example, one study in China found that the quarter of people with the highest BPA levels were almost twice as likely to have insulin resistance as those with the lowest BPA levels.

These studies do not establish that BPA actually causes insulin resistance, in either PCOS or diabetes, because it could be the case that the types of food and drinks that cause insulin resistance also happen to be the foods most contaminated with BPA. However, evidence is growing that BPA directly affects the level of insulin in the body. It appears that BPA does this by directly affecting the cells of the pancreas that release insulin.[42] BPA also reduces the production of another hormone, called adiponectin.[43] Low levels of adiponectin are closely associated with insulin resistance.

These findings suggest that BPA itself could be contributing to the widespread health problems associated with insulin resistance, such as PCOS and diabetes, as well as contributing to the fertility problems associated with these conditions.

The latest research therefore provides particularly good reasons to avoid BPA if you have PCOS or diabetes and are trying to conceive. Yet the bottom line is that anyone trying to conceive should be concerned about BPA exposure because it may disrupt hormones, contribute to chromosomal abnormalities in developing eggs, and decrease the number of eggs and the fertilization rate in women trying to conceive through IVF.

How to Avoid BPA

The good news about BPA is that there is a lot you can do to reduce your exposure, and once you take a few simple steps, the amount of BPA in your system will decrease rapidly.[44] The most important time for reducing your exposure to BPA is in the three or four months before you try to conceive, but it is never too early to start.

The first strategy to limit your exposure to BPA is to eliminate plastic from your kitchen. BPA is widely used in plastic food storage containers, bowls, and cups. When this plastic is damaged by contact with hot foods, washing in hot water, washing with harsh detergent, or heating in the microwave, it may begin to leach BPA into any food or drink it touches.[45]

When you are buying anything plastic, the most important type of plastic to stay away from is polycarbonate. This is a hard, durable plastic often marked with a seven inside the triangular recycling symbol. Polycarbonate is typically used to make reusable plastic containers. Single-use plastic water bottles are made of a different type of plastic and do not generally contain BPA.

Many kitchen products are now made with BPA-free plastic. Discarding old plastic containers and switching to these newer products is a step in the right direction. But this is not the best solution because BPA-free plastics may still leach other unknown chemicals that could be just as harmful. Companies are free to replace BPA with similar chemicals that could also disrupt hormonal systems, and there is generally no requirement for safety testing before use.

In one recent study, scientists tested more than 500 commercially available plastic food containers and found that almost all products leached chemicals having estrogen-like activity (indicating the potential to disrupt fertility), including those advertised as BPA-free. In some cases, plastic products touted as BPA-free were even worse than BPA-containing products.[46]

The researchers also found that plastics labeled "BPA-free" are particularly likely to release these other estrogenic chemicals after they have been damaged by exposure to UV light, microwaving, or moist heat. As a result, even if your plastic containers are BPA-free, the best approach is to wash them by hand in cold water and never use them with hot food or drinks. The lesson learned from BPA is that once plastic is damaged and starts to leach, it may continue to leach toxins even when it is used much later. This is exactly what happened to the laboratory mice in Dr. Hunt's experiments discussed earlier in the chapter.

Instead of switching to BPA-free plastic, a better approach is to replace plastic in your kitchen with glass, wood, stainless steel, and ceramics. This could mean replacing all your mixing bowls, storage containers, and measuring cups, but it will be a good investment for your health and for your fertility. A good place to start is with glass food storage containers because a wide range of good-quality yet inexpensive containers are available. Many brands are specifically designed to resist heat, freezing, and rapid temperature changes without breaking. These glass containers also last longer than plastic and do not absorb stains or odors the way plastic can. You can be less concerned about the plastic lids on these containers because they rarely come in close contact with food.

Another way BPA could be getting into your food is from plastic takeout containers. Be careful about regularly eating hot takeout food that comes in plastic boxes, and look for better alternatives. Studies also show that people who more frequently eat food prepared outside the home typically have higher levels of BPA exposure.[47] This is probably because restaurants are unlikely to be cautious about BPA in cans and plastic. For this reason, try to prepare more of your meals at home using fresh ingredients.

Coffee machines are another common source of BPA exposure. Automatic coffee machines typically have plastic components that come into contact with hot water or coffee, thereby leaching BPA into your coffee. If you instead make your coffee in a traditional French press, it will only come into contact with metal and glass, so you will have the best chance of toxin-free coffee.

Another important step to reducing the amount of BPA you consume is to be selective about canned foods. BPA is often used to make the lining of cans, and from there it leaches into food.[48] The amount of BPA that leaches is often particularly high if the food is acidic, such as fruit or tomatoes.[49] Another common problem is canned soup. One experiment found that consuming one can of soup from a BPA-lined can each day for five days caused a 1,000% increase in urinary BPA levels.[50]

There is, however, enormous variation between different brands and types of canned food, and some companies have switched to BPA-free cans. These companies usually proudly say so on the label. So if a can does not say "BPA-free," it is best to assume that it contains BPA. If you cannot find BPA-free canned products, the best alternative is to switch to ingredients that are fresh, dried, frozen, or packaged in glass jars.

A surprising source of BPA to be aware of is thermal paper. A little-known fact is that the paper receipts and tickets you are handed at the supermarket, movie theater, and airport can be coated with BPA.[51] A small amount can be absorbed through the skin within hours and also spreads from your hands to other objects.[52] As a result, retail employees have been shown to have very high levels of BPA in their systems.[53] The only practical way to avoid this source of BPA is to handle receipts as little as possible and wash your hands as soon as you can, particularly before eating.

Avoiding BPA takes significant effort but is worth the trouble given the likely impact on our reproductive health. That does not mean you have to become obsessed with removing BPA from your life; BPA is not the only cause of fertility issues, and restoring fertility is not as simple as avoiding BPA. But reducing your exposure is one good strategy that will likely help, particularly if you currently have a very high level in your system.

Instead of worrying about BPA on a daily basis, the best approach is to make a habit out of the simple and easy changes that make the most difference. If you have PCOS, recurrent miscarriages, or failed IVF cycles, you should be especially careful, but otherwise your goal should just be to get the level of BPA in your system well below average. This should be sufficient because it appears that what matters more than reducing BPA exposure to an extremely low level is just making sure you do not have a very high level of BPA in your system.

BPA Exposure During Pregnancy

Interestingly, the payoff for avoiding BPA does not end when you become pregnant — it is also critical for the health of your baby. Researchers have long suspected that a developing fetus is particularly vulnerable to the toxic effects of BPA.[54] It has been shown that BPA crosses the placenta from the mother's bloodstream into the baby, and BPA has been found in both the amniotic fluid and the fetus during pregnancy.[55] In fact, a fetus may be exposed to much higher levels than the pregnant mother because it is unable to metabolize BPA into harmless compounds.[56]

A large number of studies have suggested a link between exposure to BPA during pregnancy and a variety of long-term health consequences, particularly for brain development and the reproductive system.[57] In one such study, prenatal exposure was associated with behavioral abnormalities in young children.[58] While it still is not known exactly what risks BPA poses during pregnancy, getting in the habit of limiting your exposure has a dual advantage of both protecting your fertility and protecting your baby when you do become pregnant.

Action Steps
Basic, Intermediate, and *Advanced Plans*

- It is never too early to start reducing your exposure to BPA to help your future fertility.

- Reduce your exposure by:
  › Avoiding canned goods and only buying brands labeled "BPA-free."

  › Replacing plastic containers in your kitchen with glass.

  › Taking care when using plastic (even if it says "BPA-free") by washing it by hand instead of in the dishwasher and not using it with hot food or drink, or in the microwave.

  › Handling paper receipts as little as possible and washing your hands afterward.

- It is also important to continue these steps for limiting your exposure to BPA when you become pregnant to protect your growing baby.

CHAPTER 3

Phthalates and Other Toxins

"Big, sweeping life changes really boil down to small, everyday decisions."
— ALI VINCENT

BPA IS UNFORTUNATELY just one example of how chemicals that act as endocrine disruptors can stand in the way of your ability to get pregnant. Another type of toxin that may impair egg quality and fertility is a group of chemicals known as phthalates (pronounced THAL-lates).

Phthalates are widely used in soft plastic, vinyl, cleaning products, nail polish, and fragrances.[1] Just like BPA, these chemicals can compromise the activity of hormones that are critical for fertility.[2] But you can prevent this assault on your fertility by learning where phthalates may be lurking in your home and how to choose safer alternatives, giving you the best chance of getting pregnant and delivering a healthy baby.

Phthalates Are Everywhere

For decades, scientists have known that phthalates can alter the levels and activity of hormones in the body. Phthalates are now officially recognized as a reproductive toxin in the European Union,[3] and the U.S. FDA has recently acknowledged that phthalates are endocrine disruptors.[4]

As a result of these known toxic effects, certain phthalates have been banned in children's toys in Europe since 1999, and in the United States since 2008. Similar bans are also in place in Canada and Australia. As the European Commission said in 1999, the ban was intended "to protect the youngest and most vulnerable amongst us. We received scientific advice that phthalates pose a serious risk to human health."[5]

Yet if phthalates pose a serious risk to human health, why has no action been taken to ban phthalates in products other than toys? If it is beyond question that phthalates are toxic to babies and young children, why is little attention paid to the potential toxic effects before and during pregnancy?

In the words of a leading researcher in the field, Dr. Shanna Swan: "eliminating these phthalates from children's toys – I think it is important ... – but I would not do that at the expense of eliminating phthalates in products to which pregnant women are exposed. Because that is the most critical target for phthalates."[6]

Clearly any regulation that does exist is not working, because biologically active forms of phthalates have been detected in 95% of pregnant women.[7] This finding is not all that surprising given that phthalates are widely used in everything from fabric softeners to food containers to perfumes. As a result, these chemicals can be found in the bloodstream of the vast majority of people tested in the United States, Europe, and Asia.[8]

The fact that almost all women are exposed to phthalates during pregnancy is of great concern because there is strong evidence that high levels of these chemicals can negatively impact a developing fetus. The likely effects of phthalates on a fetus during pregnancy are reason enough to start to remove phthalates from your home now in order to protect your growing baby when you do become pregnant. Evidence is also emerging that high levels of phthalates may contribute to poor egg quality and therefore infertility.

Phthalates and Fertility

There are still many unknowns when it comes to the precise impact of phthalates on fertility, so it could be argued that the need to limit your exposure to phthalates while trying to conceive is unproven. Yet there is also no proof that phthalates are safe, and what little evidence we do have about the effects of phthalates is very troubling. When it comes to the impact of phthalates on health and fertility, the human population is currently participating in a grand experiment without even knowing it.

The current evidence about the impact of phthalates on fertility is based on a collection of individual studies that each tell a small part of the story rather than the large-scale human studies needed to prove a definitive impact on human fertility. Nevertheless, when added together, the current research creates a picture that is cause for concern.

The first evidence to emerge that phthalates could impact fertility came from studies showing that high doses of phthalates interfered with fertility in laboratory animals. In one of the earliest studies, rats given high doses of a particular phthalate simply stopped ovulating.[9] The phthalate used in this study, called DEHP, is the type most commonly found in soft and flexible plastic, so this discovery was quite disturbing.

Gradually the initial findings on the impact of high doses in animals were extended to show that various different phthalates have damaging effects on the human reproductive system, even at very low doses.[10] Vast amounts of animal research also show basic biological changes that likely occur in the human body, too — changes that are bad news if you are trying to have a baby.

Most studies on the harmful effects of phthalates have actually focused on male fertility, as a result of research 20 years ago showing testicular damage to newborn male rats. This early research on rats triggered several human studies, which produced substantial evidence that phthalate exposure significantly affects sperm quality, even at a low dose.[11]

While phthalates may damage sperm in a variety of ways,[12] the clearest evidence indicates that phthalates reduce sperm quality by altering hormone levels and causing oxidative stress. While sperm quality has long been the center of attention of phthalate research, and female fertility has been neglected, the latest research now indicates that phthalates harm developing eggs in much the same way.

What Happens to Eggs Exposed to Phthalates?

Whether you are trying to conceive naturally or through IVF, the ability of ovarian follicles to grow and the egg inside to mature properly is critical to fertility. In a normal ovulation cycle, one ovarian follicle matures fully and the egg inside bursts out at the time of ovulation. In a successful IVF cycle, medication stimulates a dozen or more eggs to mature at once.

Unfortunately, researchers have consistently found that phthalates significantly interfere with the growth of ovarian follicles in eggs from a variety of animals.[13] Part of the reason for this is that phthalates decrease production of estrogen by the follicles, and estrogen is one of the main drivers of follicle growth and egg development in animals and humans alike.[14]

The ability of phthalates to similarly decrease estrogen production in human follicle cells was first seen by researchers in Germany who studied the cells surrounding each egg from women undergoing IVF.[15] The actual eggs obtained in an IVF cycle were too precious to experiment on, but eggs are naturally surrounded by a layer of cells that are not needed for the rest of the IVF cycle. The researchers grew those cells in the lab with various concentrations of a phthalate, MEHP. (This is a compound produced in the body after exposure to that ubiquitous phthalate in plastic, DEHP.) They found that even at low doses, phthalate exposure suppressed the production of estrogen by the follicle cells, which would be expected to suppress follicle growth.[16]

Laboratory studies have also shown that exposure to phthalates during the time the eggs are maturing drastically interfered with egg development and the ability of eggs to fer-tilize.[17] Other studies have suggested that the impact of phthal-ates on egg development is at least partly due to a reduction in the activity of genes. Specifically, phthalates seem to impact the genes that drive meiosis and cell division that are essential for egg development.[18]

But the effect of phthalates does not end with compromising the ability of eggs to mature properly. The next critical step before pregnancy — embryo survival — could also be affected. This is a stage of conception you have probably not given much thought to unless you have been through an IVF cycle in which your fertilized embryos did not make it to the five-day mark. Unfortunately, this is not uncommon, and in a typical IVF cycle, many embryos do not survive those first few days before they are transferred to the uterus. Embryo survival is also crit-ical when trying to conceive naturally.

When animal eggs and embryos are exposed to phthalates in a laboratory, there is a clear negative effect on embryo sur-vival. Fewer embryos survive to the blastocyst stage, and at high doses, no embryos survive. [19] But this research is only very preliminary, and we do not yet know whether the same thing happens in humans at the doses we are typically exposed to in everyday life.

What we do know is that phthalates cause yet another spe-cific biological effect in humans that is very concerning for fertility. Specifically, several studies of the human population have now reported a link between phthalate exposure and increased levels of oxidative stress in the body.[20]

Oxidative stress occurs when a cell produces more reactive

oxygen molecules (commonly known as free radicals or oxidants) than it can handle. Antioxidants within the cell normally keep these reactive molecules in check, but if they cannot keep up, reactive molecules can damage the cell. This state is called oxidative stress.

Oxidative stress causes ovarian follicles to die off[21] and has been linked to the age-related decline in fertility, endometriosis, and unexplained infertility.[22] Studies have shown that exposure to phthalates may be one contributing factor to oxidative stress in developing eggs and therefore contribute to infertility.

In the largest human study on phthalates and oxidative stress, looking at data from approximately 10,000 people in the United States collected over eight years, researchers at the University of Michigan School of Public Health found that people with higher levels of several phthalates tended to have higher levels of inflammation and oxidative stress.[23]

This type of large population study can only establish a link, not a cause-and-effect relationship. But that is where animal and laboratory studies are useful because they show at a molecular level that phthalates do cause oxidative stress in a variety of cells, including eggs.

Scientists have found that phthalates cause oxidative stress by interfering with antioxidant enzymes. These enzymes are a type of defense system, there to protect cells from damage by oxidants.

Early studies found that a particular phthalate, DEHP, alters the activity of antioxidant enzymes in the liver and in the cells that produce sperm, resulting in oxidative stress.[24] In 2011, this was also shown to happen in developing eggs, indicating that oxidative stress could be responsible for at least some of the harm caused by phthalates.[25] In other words, phthalates may weaken eggs' natural antioxidant defense systems.

The implication from all these studies—that phthalates could impact IVF outcomes—was finally confirmed in 2016. In a study by Harvard researchers involving 250 women undergoing IVF, it was found that the women with higher levels of DEHP had fewer eggs retrieved and were significantly less likely to become pregnant. When compared to women with the lowest phthalate levels, those with the highest levels were 20% less likely give birth.[26]

In addition, phthalate exposure has been associated with an increased risk of endometriosis. Endometriosis is a poorly understood condition in which cells from the lining of the uterus find their way to other places in the pelvis, causing pain and impaired fertility.

Even though it is not yet known what causes endometriosis, researchers suspect that phthalate exposure could be one of many contributing factors. This is because the vast majority of studies examining this issue have shown significantly higher levels of phthalates in women with endometriosis than those without the condition.[27] In one of the largest studies to date, researchers at the National Institutes of Health, the University of Utah, and several other institutions analyzed phthalate levels in over 400 women.[28] They found a higher level of 6 different phthalate compounds in women with endometriosis. In this study, higher phthalate levels were in fact associated with a two-fold increase in the rate of endometriosis.

This by no means suggests that reducing your exposure to phthalates will improve or prevent endometriosis; we simply do not know enough to conclude that. But the research on a possible connection between phthalates and endometriosis serves as a warning to all women that phthalates could be impacting our reproductive systems in ways that are not yet understood.

Miscarriage

There is one more piece of the puzzle suggesting that phthalates may be harmful for fertility. In a small study published in 2012, women who had higher levels of a particular phthalate in their system before they became pregnant were much more likely to miscarry.[29] This study followed a group of women trying to get pregnant over six months. The researchers tested the women for the phthalate MEHP and also tested for the pregnancy hormone HCG at specific times each month. Because of this regular testing for HCG, even very early pregnancy losses were detected, including those that occurred before the women even knew they were pregnant.

The researchers found that higher levels of MEHP before pregnancy were linked to a higher rate of miscarriage. This is again just one preliminary study, but it adds further reason to be cautious of phthalates.

Phthalates During Pregnancy

While research on phthalates and female fertility is just beginning, there is much clearer evidence that unborn babies are particularly vulnerable to the toxic effects of phthalates.

Studies on how phthalates can harm a developing fetus during pregnancy have uncovered three worrisome trends: a link to premature birth, effects on the reproductive systems of baby boys, and altered brain development and behavior in early childhood.

Starting with premature birth, several studies have shown a link between exposure to phthalates during pregnancy and earlier delivery.[30] In one study led by Dr. John Meeker at the University of Michigan, together with scientists at the CDC and the Harvard School of Public Health, higher phthalate levels during the third trimester were detected in pregnant women who delivered preterm compared with those who delivered at term.[31]

One hypothesis for how phthalates could increase the risk of preterm birth is that these chemicals increase inflammation, which raises the risk of earlier labor.[32] It is also plausible that phthalates, which we know alter hormone levels in the ovaries, may contribute to preterm birth by lowering the levels of estrogen and progesterone in the uterus.[33]

Another troubling effect of phthalates during pregnancy is sometimes described as "demasculinization" of boys. One of the pioneers in this field is Dr. Shanna Swan, Professor of Preventive Medicine at Mount Sinai Hospital in New York. In 2005 and 2008, she published the results of groundbreaking research showing that women with higher levels of certain phthalates during pregnancy were more likely to have baby boys with specific problems with their reproductive systems.[34]

Several years earlier, a similar effect of phthalates during pregnancy had been seen in mice and rats by many different researchers. A characteristic set of changes in these animals had even become known as "phthalate syndrome."[35] This syndrome included incomplete testicular descent and several other specific genital malformations. While phthalate syndrome was of great concern, no one really knew the implications for humans exposed to these same chemicals.

There was some hope that phthalate syndrome was limited to high-dose exposure and lab animals, but Dr. Swan quashed those hopes with definitive research showing that a similar thing was happening in people, and at the doses many women are exposed to on a daily basis.[36] As Dr. Swan explained, "we were the first to show a link between prenatal phthalate exposure and reproductive development in humans."[37]

The consensus among scientists now studying how phthalates interfere with male reproductive development is that phthalates suppress the production of testosterone in male fetuses during pregnancy.[38] Numerous animal studies have concluded that phthalates interfere with testosterone production in male fetuses,[39] and testosterone is critical to development of the male reproductive system.

Many different research groups have also found a strong link between exposure to phthalates during pregnancy and altered brain development and behavior in babies and children. For example, in one recent study of 319 pregnant women conducted by the Columbia Center for Children's Environmental Health in New York, researchers measured phthalate levels in each mother's system during pregnancy.[40] Then three years later, the researchers assessed the toddlers' mental development and motor skills, and noted any behavioral problems.

The results were disconcerting: Children whose mothers had higher levels of phthalates in their system while pregnant scored significantly lower on measures of mental, motor, and behavioral development.

This finding was unfortunately not new. Many other studies had also reached the same conclusion.[41] Researchers have hypothesized that this impact on brain development could be due to the effects of phthalates on thyroid hormones. This theory is supported by research consistently demonstrating that phthalates interfere with thyroid function, [42] and the critical role the thyroid plays in brain development,[43] including during pregnancy.[44]

Phthalates have also been found to contribute to allergies and eczema in children,[45] and there is a clear link between living in a home with phthalate-laden plastic flooring and an increased risk of asthma in children.[46] Babies are often exposed to much higher levels of certain phthalates because they teethe on plastic and absorb phthalates through their skin from baby care products such as shampoos and lotions.[47]

Researchers have found that the more baby care products mothers use on their infants (such as shampoos, lotions, and powders), the more phthalates are found in the babies' systems.[48]

Fortunately, this exposure of your eggs, your developing fetus, and your newborn baby to toxic levels of phthalates is not inevitable. You can do quite a few simple things to reduce the level of phthalates in your body and in your home.

Reducing Your Exposure to Phthalates

The first place to look when trying to remove phthalates from your home is your bathroom. Cosmetics and personal care products such as hairspray, lotions, fragrances, and nail polish often have very high levels of phthalates. These chemicals can be absorbed through the skin from lotions[49] or inhaled from products that are sprayed into the air. Phthalates can in fact be found in almost anything fragranced. As a result, it is not surprising that women typically have higher levels than men of the types of phthalates used in cosmetics and personal care products.[50]

Nail polish often has a higher concentration of phthalates than any other cosmetic product; this is reason enough to stop wearing nail polish while trying to conceive. Nail polish also often contains other nasty chemicals such as formaldehyde and toluene, both of which have been linked to reduced fertility and increased risk of miscarriage.[51] Many different studies across the world have concluded that women exposed to formaldehyde on a daily basis through their workplace (nail salons, hospitals, and laboratories) have more than twice the chance of miscarriage. [52]

Major nail polish companies recently agreed to remove this "toxic trio" of formaldehyde, toluene, and the specific phthalate DBP from their products, labeling the new formulations "three-free." However in 2012, a study by the California EPA found that many nail products claiming to be "three-free" still had one or more of these dangerous chemicals, sometimes at very high levels.

Buying nail polish labeled "three-free" and "phthalate-free" is a safer option than traditional formulations, but in the end we may not be able to trust what manufacturers say. The best brands are probably those sold at health food stores and ranked as less toxic by the Environmental Working Group Skin Deep Cosmetics Database, such as Honeybee Gardens. If you cannot bear to part with traditional nail polish, the danger may be minimized by ensuring good ventilation during your manicure.

You can sometimes recognize phthalates in lotions and other cosmetic products by their chemical names and abbreviations. Occasionally you will see the word "phthalate" buried in a long chemical name, such as di-n-butylphthalate (DBP) or diethyl phthalate (DEP), listed in the ingredients of deodorant, perfume, hair products, and moisturizers.

But phthalates are often present without being identified anywhere on the label. Companies are allowed to do this because of a loophole whereby manufacturers are not required to identify individual ingredients in fragrances. Anytime you see the word "fragrance" in a list of ingredients, you can assume that the product likely contains phthalates.

If you wear perfume on a daily basis, this is likely to be another one of the main sources of toxic phthalates in your body. [53] Studies have found that women who wear perfume can have double the concentration of some phthalates in their system. Perfumes are also a cocktail of dozens of other chemicals that can potentially cause allergies and disrupt hormones, many of which have never been tested for safety. If you cannot give up fragrance altogether, consider switching to all-natural fragrances or body lotions scented with natural essential oils and labeled as "phthalate-free."

Another place to look for phthalates is anything made out of soft plastic such as PVC (polyvinylchloride), often called vinyl. This type of plastic is used to make shower curtains, raincoats, yoga mats, school supplies, place mats, and makeup bags. In fact, if a plastic product is flexible, it probably contains phthalates unless the label specifically says it does not. From these products, the phthalates can be released into the air and inhaled, or released into food.[54]

Because phthalates are found in so many products, reducing the amount you are exposed to can seem like an overwhelming project. But an easy way to start is to remove some of the worst offenders in your home, then over time replace other phthalate-laden products as needed. For example, you may decide to stop using air fresheners, nail polish, and perfume. This is a particularly powerful first step because these products are typically highest in toxic phthalates.[55]

You could also switch to laundry detergents, fabric softeners, and cleaning supplies that are made with only plant-based natural ingredients or specifically labeled as phthalate free (such as those made by The Honest Company and Seventh Generation). Those simple steps alone could make an enormous difference to your level of phthalate exposure.

If you want to take the next step, you could replace your hair-care and skin-care products with fragrance-free products or ones specifically labeled as "phthalate free" (such as those made by The Honest Company and Avalon Organics). For up-to-date product recommendations see www.itstartswiththeegg.com

The most important skin-care product to replace is probably your body lotion because it is applied over a greater surface area, so you are likely to absorb more chemicals through your skin.

You may also want to consider replacing your vinyl shower curtain with one made from nylon, cotton, or polyester, and replacing your yoga mat with one labeled "PVC free" (Gaiam is just one company now making these less toxic yoga mats).

The final step in your program to reduce phthalates in your home may be to limit the amount of packaged, processed food you buy. Food is actually a major source of phthalates because phthalates enter the food chain at every stage, from growing livestock and spraying pesticides on fruit and vegetables to processing, packaging, and commercial food preparation.[56] For this reason, phthalates are commonly found in even the healthiest foods.[57]

There is no foolproof way to escape phthalates in food, but the best strategy is likely to be to avoid highly processed food, avoid food packaged or stored in plastic, and choose organic fruits, vegetables, and meats.

When five families in San Francisco were given a diet strictly applying this strategy for several days, their levels of certain phthalate metabolites fell by over 50%.[58] These families had meals prepared for them – almost exclusively using fresh, organic ingredients. The meals were also prepared and stored without plastic utensils or containers, and the participants were only allowed to drink coffee made in a French press or ceramic drip rather than a coffee machine with plastic parts inside. It may not be practical to follow these rules every day, but this study suggests that any reduction of packaged food in favor of organic produce and meat is likely to help reduce phthalate levels, along with having many other nutritional benefits.

Choosing organic produce is a particularly powerful way of reducing your toxin exposure because doing so avoids the phthalates and many other hormone-disrupting chemicals found in pesticides. (Phthalates have long been used as solvents in pesticides, although many specific phthalates have recently been removed from the EPA's list of approved pesticide ingredients.)

Avoiding food packaged in clear plastic is another great step to take because packaging such as clamshells and blister packs are often made from phthalate-laden PVC, which can be identified by the number 3 in the recycling symbol. While most plastic bottles used for water, soda, and condiments are made from a type of plastic called PET or PETE, which in theory is not manufactured using phthalates, researchers have consistently found that water packaged in these plastic bottles contains much higher phthalate levels than water packaged in glass bottles, perhaps because of contamination during plastic recycling.[59]

It is difficult to completely avoid buying food and drinks packaged in plastic, but whenever you have a choice between glass and plastic, choose glass, and look for opportunities to replace plastic-packaged foods when you can. A 2013 study by researchers at New York University found that children who ate more fruit had lower phthalate levels, whereas greater meat, fish, and poultry consumption was associated with higher phthalate levels.[60]

It is up to you to decide which changes are easiest for you to make and how careful you want to be. Any of these steps will help and will not only reduce your exposure to phthalates but will probably also reduce your exposure to a host of other potentially toxic chemicals. This is because plastics made from PVC can leach lead and cadmium,[61] while cosmetics that contain phthalates often also contain other harmful chemicals such as parabens.

In one recent study, Harvard researchers suggested that propyl-paraben, a common cosmetic ingredient, is linked to diminished ovarian reserve.[62] Cosmetics companies that go to the trouble of eliminating phthalates from their products are more likely to stay away from these other harmful chemicals, too.

All these steps to minimizing phthalate exposure while trying to conceive will have the added benefit of reducing phthalate levels in your home when you do become pregnant and will protect your unborn baby from the multitude of health risks posed by phthalate exposure in utero and during early child-hood. Yet preparing to bring your baby home will pose an addi-tional challenge when it comes to avoiding phthalates because baby products are a surprising source of toxic phthalates.

In addition to all the fragranced baby shampoos and lotions that contain phthalates, just about every company that makes crib mattresses, mattress pads, and changing pads uses PVC as a waterproof layer, despite the well-known health dangers. Many companies also package baby clothes, sheets, and blan-kets in this plastic, allowing these nasty chemicals to get into the fabric.

The fact that phthalates are banned in children's toys but widely used in baby products is perplexing and will hopefully change soon. In the meantime, one company that makes good-quality crib mattresses, changing pads, and other excellent baby products without this toxic plastic is Naturepedic. The Honest Company and California Baby also make phthalate-free shampoos and baby lotions.

The world is also full of many other toxins, but in general we know very little about how they affect fertility. There is clear evidence that BPA and phthalates have the potential to disrupt hormones and therefore compromise fertility and early childhood development. Unfortunately, many other toxins in our environment are suspected of doing the same, but the research on how these other toxins impact fertility is just beginning.

If you want to be particularly cautious and minimize exposure to other known hormone disruptors, the best place to start is the Environmental Working Group's dirty dozen list of endocrine disruptors.[63] In addition to BPA and phthalates, this list contains ten other common toxins that you can avoid in surprisingly simple ways:

Dioxin: Choose low-fat meat and dairy, and use olive oil instead of butter.

Atrazine: Buy organic fruit and vegetables, and use a water filter certified to remove atrazine (see the Environmental Working Group's Water Filter Buying Guide[64]).

Perchlorate: Although difficult to avoid, you can minimize its potential to disrupt thyroid hormones by getting enough iodine in your diet, such as through iodized salt.

Fire Retardants: Air out your home and vacuum regularly with a HEPA-filtered vacuum cleaner.

Lead: Buy a water filter certified to remove lead, and take off your shoes at the door.

Arsenic: Use a water filter certified to remove arsenic.

Mercury: Choose low-mercury fish, and don't handle the new compact-fluorescent light bulbs. If dropped and broken, these bulbs release mercury vapors into the air.

Perfluorinated Chemicals (PFCs): Use stainless steel and cast iron cookware instead of nonstick pans.

Organophosphate Pesticides: Buy organic fruit and vegetables if you can, or choose varieties less likely to be contaminated with high levels of pesticides – typically those with a protective outer peel, such as pineapple, mangoes, kiwi, corn, cabbage, and avocado.

Glycol Ethers: Avoid cleaning products containing 2-butoxyethanol (EGBE) and methoxydiglycol (DEGME).

In addition, new evidence is emerging that a group of chemicals called quaternary ammonium compounds may pose a serious threat to fertility while dramatically increasing the risk of birth defects.[65] These chemicals are used in many disinfectant sprays and wipes (including certain Lysol and Clorox products). While the danger of quaternary ammonium compounds is only just beginning to come to light, the research in this area further emphasizes the need to choose natural, non-toxic household products rather than gambling with the dozens of untested chemicals found in conventional products.

As Dr. Swan explained, "I think we have now a lot of data that environmental chemicals can and do lower sperm count, impact time to conception, increase fetal loss in early pregnancy, affect pregnancy outcomes. Do we need more studies? Of course we do. But do we have enough information to act on these studies that we have? I say that we do."[66]

Further Reading

- Pass Up the Poison Plastic, the PVC-Free Guide for Your Family and Home. Center for Health, Environment and Justice.

- Environmental Working Group Guide to Healthy Cleaning (http://www.ewg.org /guides/cleaners)

- Environmental Working Group Skin Deep Cosmetic Database (http://www.ewg.org/skindeep)

Action Steps
Basic, Intermediate, and *Advanced Plans*

- Reduce phthalate exposure from cosmetics by replacing hair-care and skin-care products with ones labeled fragrance-free or, better yet, phthalate-free. Detailed product recommendations are available at www.itstartswiththeegg.com

- Try to avoid using perfume, hair spray, and nail polish.

- Look for cleaning and laundry products that are plant-based, fragrance-free, or phthalate-free.

- Consider whether there is anything in your home made out of soft, flexible plastic, such vinyl or PVC, that can be replaced with a safer alternative.

- Reduce your phthalate exposure from food by choosing fresh, unprocessed food and generally minimizing contact with plastic.

CHAPTER 4

Unexpected Obstacles to Fertility

"Discovery consists of seeing what everybody has seen and thinking what nobody has thought."
— ALBERT SZENT-GYORGYI

I F YOU ARE having trouble conceiving or have had one or more miscarriages, you should ask your doctor to test you for several easily treated conditions that are often missed: vitamin D deficiency, underactive thyroid, and celiac disease. Not all doctors will think about testing for these conditions unless you ask, but each condition has a surprisingly strong link to infertility and miscarriage. Any one of these factors could be the missing link in your treatment plan and, once corrected, will give you the best chance of a healthy pregnancy.

Surprising Factor 1: Vitamin D

In the past decade, vitamin D has become a hot area of research; low levels of vitamin D have now been implicated in a wide variety of diseases, including diabetes, cancer, obesity, multiple sclerosis, and arthritis. Although the research on the role of vitamin D and fertility has only just begun and is somewhat inconsistent,[1] several studies indicate that low levels of vitamin D may negatively impact fertility.

In one of the most compelling studies, which was published in 2012, researchers at Columbia University and the University of Southern California (USC) measured vitamin D levels in nearly 200 women undergoing IVF. Of the Caucasian women in the group, the odds of pregnancy were *four times* higher for women with high vitamin D levels compared to those with a vitamin D deficiency.[2] This trend was not seen in women of Asian ethnicity, but for Caucasian women there was such a powerful difference in the chance of becoming pregnant that it should make anyone about to go through IVF think twice about their own vitamin D levels.

The link between higher pregnancy rates and high vitamin D levels seen in the Columbia/USC study is consistent with a previous similar study in Turkey. That study found that in the group of women with the highest vitamin D levels, 47% became pregnant, while among women with low vitamin D levels, the pregnancy rate was only 20%.[3] Another more recent IVF study revealed a higher fertilization and implantation rate in a group of women with higher vitamin D levels.[4]

It is not yet known how vitamin D is involved in fertility, but researchers suspect that one of the ways it may improve fertility is by making the uterine lining more receptive to pregnancy.[5] Research also indicates that vitamin D plays a role in hormone production, including production of hormones that control reproduction. Specifically, some scientists think that vitamin D deficiency may contribute to infertility by interrupting the estrogen system and also reducing production of antimullerian hormone (AMH), which is involved in the growth of ovarian follicles.[6] Another enticing clue about the role of vitamin D in fertility is the discovery that there are specific receptors for vitamin D in cells in the ovaries and the uterus.[7]

It is likely that vitamin D supplements can only improve fertility if you are currently deficient, but a deficiency is surprisingly common, particularly in cooler climates. By some estimates, as much as 36% of the U.S. population is deficient,[8] and the rate nearly doubled from 1994 to 2004.[9] Researchers believe this is largely due to reduced time outdoors and greater use of sunscreen because even though we obtain small amounts from food, the vast majority of vitamin D in the body is made after the skin is exposed to sunlight.[10] In fact, the decrease in fertility rates during winter is thought to be caused by a reduction in vitamin D levels.[11]

Vitamin D deficiency is also especially common in women with PCOS. One study in Scotland found a severe vitamin D deficiency in 44% of women with PCOS but in just 11% of those without the condition.[12] The same study found a link between lower vitamin D levels and the degree of insulin resistance. In other words, women more deficient in vitamin D had more significant metabolic imbalances.

This same link between lower vitamin D levels and the

specific hormonal imbalances in PCOS has been found in several other studies.[13] Thus, researchers suspect that low vitamin D levels may contribute to insulin resistance and other hormonal imbalances that cause infertility in PCOS. If this is true, vitamin D supplements may correct some of these hormonal imbalances and improve fertility.

Further research has provided some initial evidence that correcting vitamin D deficiency can improve PCOS. For example, a study in Austria found that 50% of women with PCOS treated with vitamin D for 6 months had improved ovulation. Vitamin D supplements also decreased glucose levels and rebalanced hormones.[14]

While we await further research to clarify the exact value of vitamin D supplements in treating infertility, if you are having difficulty conceiving (with or without PCOS), it is probably a good idea to ask your doctor to test your vitamin D levels.

If you do have a deficiency, it can easily be corrected with a daily supplement. Many doctors will recommend at least 2,000 international units (IU) of vitamin D per day, but you should follow your doctor's recommendation as to the specific dose to take.

Regardless of the dose, to obtain the most benefit from a vitamin D supplement, it is important to choose one that is formulated in an oil capsule, rather than a solid tablet, and to take it with a meal containing some fat. Both measures significantly improve the absorption of vitamin D because it is a fat-soluble vitamin.[15]

Alternatively, you can boost your vitamin D levels naturally by spending more time outside in the sun, although this is difficult in winter months, and sun damage to skin is still a concern. You can also get some vitamin D from foods such as fish, eggs, and fortified milk, but you will probably not be able to correct a deficiency with food sources alone. If you have a vitamin D deficiency, a supplement may be the best way to improve your chances of getting pregnant.

Surprising Factor 2: Hypothyroidism

If you have been struggling with infertility or miscarriages, you should also ask your doctor to check your thyroid hormone and antibody levels. Even very mild thyroid conditions can dramatically increase the risk of miscarriage. In addition, hypothyroidism (underactive thyroid) is common in women with premature ovarian failure, unexplained infertility, and ovulation disorders.

The link between miscarriage and thyroid disorders was discovered by accident more than 20 years ago. The research project that uncovered the link was originally designed to understand why some women develop thyroid disorders after they give birth. To investigate this, more than 500 women in New York were screened for thyroid hormones and thyroid antibodies in the first trimester of pregnancy. Thyroid antibodies were tested because their presence is a sign that the immune system is mounting an attack on the thyroid, which is the most common cause of hypothyroidism.[16]

As this study unfolded, the researchers noticed a high number of miscarriages in the women who tested positive for thyroid antibodies. The researchers decided to look at the miscarriage rates more closely and found that in women with thyroid antibodies, the miscarriage rate more than doubled.[17] This finding was so unexpected that the researchers were not sure whether the results showed a real link or just reflected a statistical fluke.[18]

In the 20 years since that initial research, dozens of studies have confirmed that having an autoimmune thyroid disorder significantly increases the risk of miscarriage. In a large study in Pakistan published in 2006, the miscarriage rate was even higher than earlier studies suggested — 36% in women who tested thyroid antibody positive compared to just 1.8% for those without thyroid antibodies.[19]

Thyroid conditions are also extremely common in women with recurrent miscarriage — typically defined as women who have lost 3 or more pregnancies. Thyroid antibodies are present in more than a third of women with recurrent miscarriage, compared to 7–13% of women without a history of miscarriage.[20]

Doctors are not entirely sure why thyroid antibodies pose such a problem in early pregnancy. One of the most puzzling facts is that having antibodies against the thyroid increases the miscarriage risk significantly, even when the thyroid is still functioning well and thyroid hormone levels are basically normal.[21] In these cases, researchers believe thyroid antibodies may contribute to miscarriage risk by reducing the ability of the thyroid to rise to the demand of making extra hormones during pregnancy. That is, even when the thyroid is functioning normally before pregnancy, thyroid autoimmunity may result in a small decrease in the ability of the thyroid to function, which can be very detrimental in early pregnancy.

Even though thyroid antibodies do raise miscarriage rates in women without any obvious decline in thyroid function, the miscarriage rate is especially high when tests show that in addition to thyroid antibodies, the hormone levels are abnormal because the thyroid is struggling to keep up.[22] Researchers have found that the miscarriage rate is 69% higher in women with a clearly underactive thyroid gland and hormonal imbalances.[23]

This, believe it or not, is good news because a firm link between the disruption of thyroid hormones and miscarriage implies that correcting thyroid hormone levels may also help prevent miscarriage. Just as we would hope, initial research shows that thyroid hormone treatment is incredibly effective at reducing miscarriage rates.

For example, a study in Italy of women with untreated thyroid antibodies found a miscarriage rate of 13.8% compared to 2.4% in women without thyroid problems. But when women with thyroid antibodies received thyroid hormone treatments during pregnancy, the miscarriage rate dropped to just 3.5% — much lower than untreated women and approaching that of women without any thyroid problems.[24] These positive results have been seen in several other studies,[25] providing powerful evidence that treating hypothyroidism can make a significant difference to miscarriage rates.

Thyroid disorders are, however, not just related to miscarriage — they are also very common in women with unexplained infertility, ovulation disorders, and premature ovarian failure.

Premature ovarian failure is a condition in which the number and quality of eggs severely limits fertility. IVF is often the only path to becoming pregnant in women with this diagnosis, and even then the success rates are very low. Cycles are often canceled because not enough eggs grow and mature in response to stimulation medication. Premature ovarian failure is poorly understood, but one factor that has recently emerged is the link to thyroid disorders.

It has become apparent that even a very mild reduction in thyroid activity, a condition called "subclinical" hypothyroidism, could be a major contributor to premature ovarian failure. In recent studies, while only 4% of healthy women were found to have subclinical hypothyroidism, the rate increased to 15% of women with ovulatory infertility and 40% of women with premature ovarian failure.[26]

Another study demonstrated that 20% of women with ovulation disorders have subclinical hypothyroidism, finding that this condition is more than twice as common in women with ovulation disorders as in women with normal ovulation (20.5% versus 8.3%).[27]

As with miscarriage rates, the results of treatment with thyroid hormones are very encouraging. In one such study, after infertile women with subclinical hypothyroidism were treated with the synthetic thyroid hormone levothyroxine, 44% of the women became pregnant.[28] Studies have also shown that treating mild thyroid conditions can increase the number of good-quality embryos in IVF.[29]

Thyroid antibodies are also very common in PCOS, with studies finding these antibodies in a quarter of women with PCOS.[30] Women with PCOS are also more likely to have hormonal imbalances indicative of underactive thyroid.

If you have a history of miscarriage, PCOS, unexplained infertility, an ovulation disorder, or premature ovarian failure, you should insist on thyroid testing — including thyroid antibodies, not just hormone levels. If a problem is detected, talk to your doctor about the critical need for effective treatment to help you become pregnant and prevent miscarriage. If your doctor does not appreciate the importance of carefully managing hypothyroidism in the context of infertility and miscarriage (and some may not), get a second opinion.

Surprising Factor 3: Celiac Disease

Another factor that can contribute to infertility is celiac disease. This is a relatively common immune disorder in which gluten triggers the immune system to wage war on the body. The most well-known symptoms of celiac disease mimic irritable bowel syndrome, but the vast majority of people with this condition do not actually show these classic gastrointestinal symptoms.[31] Celiac disease can also manifest as anemia, headaches, fatigue, joint pain, skin disorders such as psoriasis, and a variety of other symptoms that differ widely between people.

Because celiac disease affects everyone differently, the condition often goes undiagnosed for many years. In Italy, celiac disease is taken very seriously, and all children are routinely screened for the disease by age 6. But in the rest of the world, people with celiac disease often endure symptoms for many years before finding out the cause. By some reports, the average person with celiac disease visits 5 or more doctors before they are finally diagnosed, and in the United States it takes an average of 5-11 years to get a diagnosis.[32] Meanwhile, under the surface the immune system is waging war on the body, causing inflammation and damage.

One of the hallmarks of celiac disease is that the immune

system severely damages the lining of the intestines, which in turn prevents proper absorption of nutrients. This inability to absorb nutrients leads to vitamin and mineral deficiencies that contribute to infertility.[33]

The link between celiac disease and infertility was first suggested in 1982,[34] but even now many doctors do not think to test for celiac disease in women with unexplained infertility. This is unfortunate because the data show that celiac disease is very common in women with unexplained infertility and that fertility improves once the condition is treated.

Specifically, research in performed in Italy, India, and Brazil suggests that celiac disease is approximately three times more common in women with unexplained infertility than in the general population.[35] In the United States, a small initial study found no link between celiac disease and unexplained infertility,[36] but later studies, including one performed by Columbia University and Mayo Clinic, have found a significantly higher rate of celiac disease in women with unexplained infertility.[37]

Miscarriages are also very common in women with untreated celiac disease. One group of researchers found the miscarriage rate in women with untreated celiac disease to be almost nine times higher than in treated celiac patients.[38] The fact that women with "treated celiac disease," which involves carefully following a gluten-free diet, had a much lower miscarriage rate is very encouraging, showing that it is possible to reduce your risk of miscarriage if you have celiac disease.

A significant proportion of celiacs also have elevated levels of a specific type of antibody known to cause miscarriage (antiphospholipid antibodies), but anecdotal reports suggest that these antibodies decline dramatically after adopting a strict gluten-free diet.[39] This is exactly what happened to one 34-year-old woman with antiphospholipid syndrome who suffered two miscarriages. Once diagnosed with celiac disease, she began a gluten-free diet, and within 6 months the previously elevated antibodies were undetectable.[40]

Putting all the research together, in an average group of 20 women with unexplained infertility, we would expect that 1 or 2 of those women will have celiac disease, which could be a major factor in their infertility. Finding out if you are one of those women affected by the condition could be very valuable in your quest to become pregnant.

Research also clearly establishes that if you do have celiac disease, following a strict gluten-free diet is imperative. One example of how a gluten-free diet could improve fertility comes from studies showing that previously disrupted menstrual cycles often return to normal once a gluten-free diet is adopted. Research has found that more than a third of women with untreated celiac disease have amenorrhea, which means that menstrual periods sometimes stop for months at a time. After following a gluten-free diet, this condition often resolves itself.[41]

One of the ways celiac disease is believed to contribute to infertility is by interfering with absorption of folic acid and other vitamins.[42] Low folate levels then contribute to high homocysteine levels. In people with untreated celiac disease, it is very common to see high levels of homocysteine and low levels of folate,[43] both of which are strongly linked to poor egg quality, infertility, and high miscarriage rates.[44]

Excluding gluten is likely to improve fertility in women

with celiac disease because it allows the lining of the intestines to heal and restores the body's ability to absorb vital nutrients. Just as we would hope, it appears that strictly following a gluten-free diet helps bring homocysteine and folate levels back to normal.[45]

Some researchers have found, however, that up to half of celiac patients carefully treated with a gluten-free diet still showed vitamin deficiencies. Specifically, many people with celiac disease who have followed a gluten-free diet for many years still have lower levels of folate and vitamin B6 and high levels of homocysteine.[46] But it appears that the situation can be improved with vitamin supplements.

When a large group of people with celiac disease were given a daily dose of folic acid, vitamin B12, and vitamin B6 for six months, their homocysteine levels returned to normal, and they reported significant improvements in well-being compared to those given a placebo.[47] This is not to say that a gluten-free diet should be ignored in favor of supplements, because celiac disease causes many other problems in addition to vitamin deficiencies, but rather suggests that prenatal vitamin supplements are likely to be even more important for people with celiac disease.

If you have any symptoms of celiac disease, including stomach pain, irritable bowel syndrome, fatigue, psoriasis, anemia, or chronic joint pain, ask your doctor to test you for celiac disease. Even if you do not have any of these symptoms but have a history of unexplained infertility or unexplained miscarriage, you should also ask to be tested for celiac disease just in case you are one of the many people in whom this condition contributes to infertility but causes no other outward symptoms.

Celiac disease also has a very significant genetic component, so if anyone in your family has celiac disease, there is very good reason to be tested, even if you have no symptoms.

While your doctor may not be familiar enough with the research to be particularly receptive to testing for celiac disease solely on the basis of unexplained infertility, this approach is supported by the researchers who know the most about the link between celiac disease and infertility. The researchers at the Columbia University Celiac Disease Center and Mayo Clinic who published one of the key studies on this topic have suggested that "it may now be reasonable to screen any patient presenting with unexplained infertility, regardless of the absence or presence of gastrointestinal symptoms."[48]

If you do have celiac disease, strictly following a gluten-free diet could greatly improve your fertility and reduce your risk of miscarriage. This will mean carefully avoiding any food containing wheat, rye, or barley and anything that could be contaminated with even small amounts of these grains.

It is a difficult lifestyle adjustment, but gluten-free products are becoming more widely available. Although following a gluten-free diet will be very important to your fertility if you have celiac disease, it is not the only step to take. You will also have a greater need for vitamin supplements, so a daily prenatal multivitamin will be essential. This combination of strictly adhering to a gluten-free diet and taking a daily prenatal vitamin is likely to make you feel much better, improve your fertility, and reduce your miscarriage risk. But the only way to know whether this will help you is to first be tested for celiac disease.

As a side note, it is now thought that 30–40% of people with celiac disease will also have a thyroid disorder, and celiac disease brings a threefold higher chance of developing thyroid disease.[49] As a practical matter, this means that if you have been found to have either thyroid disease or celiac disease, there is even more reason for your doctor to check for the other condition if you are struggling with infertility or miscarriage.

Surprising Factor 4: Dental Care

Yet another surprising factor that may impact your chance of conceiving and carrying to term is the health of your gums. For several years, researchers have seen evidence that gum disease significantly increases the risk of preterm birth and low birth weight.[50] A study published in the *Journal of the American Dental Association* reported that women with an advanced form of gum disease, called periodontitis, are 4–7 times more likely to deliver prematurely.[51] Periodontitis also increases the risk of miscarriage. [52]

Gum disease is caused by bacteria building up between the teeth and gums, causing soreness and sometimes bleeding. The most common form of gum disease, called gingivitis, affects nearly half of women of childbearing age. If left untreated, this can progress to periodontitis, in which the gums start to pull away from the teeth, creating spaces called periodontal pockets that become infected. The infection causes an immune response that can result in inflammation spreading into the circulatory system.

The relationship between gum disease and miscarriage or premature birth is thought to be due to either the systemic inflammation that results from the bacterial infection or, alternatively, the bacteria from the gums making their way into amniotic fluid and causing a local immune response, which in turn increases the risk of miscarriage or premature birth.[53]

Yet the impact of gum disease does not end with miscarriage and premature birth — it may also increase the time it takes to get pregnant in the first place. This unexpected link was first revealed in 2011 by Dr. Roger Hart and a team of researchers at the University of Western Australia. As part of a larger study aiming to find out whether treating periodontal disease could improve pregnancy outcomes, the researchers screened more than three thousand pregnant women for periodontal disease, along with collecting information about how long it took each woman to conceive.[54]

The researchers found that on average, the women with periodontal disease took 2 months longer to conceive. Nearly a quarter of Caucasian women and 40% of non-Caucasian women were found to have periodontal disease, and these women took on average 7 months to conceive, compared to 5 months for women without gum disease. Gum disease was also much more common in the women who had taken more than a year to conceive. As Dr. Hart suggested, these significant results indicate that all women should get a dental checkup before trying to conceive.

While it does not take much to get gum disease, it is also easy to prevent and reverse with regular flossing, brushing, and professional dental cleanings. Even fairly advanced periodontal disease can usually be resolved after less than four treatments by a periodontist.[55]

Action Steps

Basic, Intermediate, and Advanced Plans

If you have had difficulty getting pregnant or have lost one or more pregnancies to miscarriage, ask your doctor to test you for vitamin D deficiency, thyroid disease, and celiac disease. You should also get a dental checkup for gum disease. Any one of these easily treatable conditions could be standing in the way of your ability to have a baby.

Part 2

How to Choose the **Right** **Supplements**

CHAPTER 5

Prenatal Multivitamins

"The more original a discovery, the more obvious it seems afterwards."

— ARTHUR KOESTLER

Recommended for:
Basic, Intermediate, and *Advanced Fertility Plans*

TAKING A PRENATAL multivitamin every day is one of the most important things you can do to prepare for pregnancy. And it is never too early to start. Vitamins such as folate are not only critical to preventing birth defects but may also make it easier to get pregnant in the first place by restoring ovulation and boosting egg quality. Surprisingly, some vitamins can also reduce the risk of miscarriage. For all these reasons, it is important to start taking your prenatal vitamin early — if possible, at least three months before trying to conceive.

Folate

Folate is a B vitamin needed throughout the body for hundreds of different biological processes. Folic acid is the synthetic form of folate used in supplements. This important vitamin is traditionally known for its role in preventing serious birth defects such as spina bifida, but recent research has also uncovered new evidence that folate plays a significant role even earlier – during the development of the egg. Because eggs begin maturing three to four months before ovulation, this suggests that the earlier you can start taking folate, the better.

It is not at all surprising that folate impacts egg quality, because it is important for making new copies of DNA, such as when a cell divides, and for making the building blocks of proteins. Both of these processes play enormous roles in early egg and embryo development. Before delving into the research showing that folic acid boosts fertility, it is useful to understand the broader context of how folic acid came to be such an important part of planning for pregnancy.

Folic acid supplementation has now been hailed as one of the greatest public health achievements of the late 20th century.[1] Yet it was not always so, and early research into the role of folic acid in preventing birth defects was marred by controversy. This controversy furnishes interesting background information for the other supplements discussed in this book because it provides an example of why there is often a huge gap between research findings and medical practice.

Until the 1990s, doctors had very little understanding of what could be done to prevent neural tube defects, which often resulted in stillbirth, death shortly after birth, or lifelong paralysis.

The world changed in 1991, when researchers in England published the results of a large study showing that 70–80% of neural tube defects could be prevented by taking a folic acid supplement immediately before pregnancy.[2] The beneficial effects of folic acid were so clear that the study was actually halted early so that more women could benefit from the findings.

Yet this large study was not the first to reveal that folic acid supplements could prevent neural tube defects. An earlier study showing the same thing,[3] published in 1981, generated many years of hostile criticism.[4]

The criticism mainly centered on the design of the trial because folic acid was given to all women presenting with a history of a previous pregnancy affected by neural tube defects, and the control group consisted of women who were already pregnant at the time they came to the doctors running the study. This is a departure from the ideal study design, in which a group of women are randomly assigned to receive either folic acid or a placebo, and the doctor and patient are "blind" as to which pill is being taken until the data are analyzed. This is referred to as a "gold standard" clinical trial and is designed to minimize the effect of bias.

In the case of folic acid, it was another 10 years before the results of the 1991 randomized, double-blind, placebo-controlled trial were available to confirm the initial research findings. In the meantime, the authors of the first study claimed that their results were persistently ignored while the possibility of a bias was overemphasized.[5] The practical impact of this controversy is that between 1981, when there was very good evidence of the protective effects of folic acid, and 1991, when a double-blind, placebo-controlled study finally satisfied the skeptics, 10 years passed, during which time many women who should have been taking folic acid supplements were not, likely resulting in countless tragic outcomes that could have been prevented.

This serves as a cautionary tale that we should not overlook the best available evidence while we wait for the perfect clinical study — a philosophy echoed throughout this book. This philosophy of acting on the "best evidence" does of course need to be limited by safety concerns. If the benefit of a supplement is clear but we do not yet have reliable evidence of safety, it is absolutely necessary to wait for further research. But if safety has been firmly established in good-quality studies and there is good, but not perfect, evidence of a very significant benefit, we have every reason to act rather than waiting for a perfect clinical study that may never happen.

This is particularly true in the fertility context, in which women may have only one or two chances to conceive with IVF before running out of financial (or emotional) resources, and there is often no time to wait. That is the background for the supplement recommendations in the rest of this book: weighing all the available evidence for each supplement rather than waiting for medical practice to catch up with research.

Returning to the specific example of folic acid, we now know that taking this supplement before pregnancy dramatically cuts the risk of spina bifida and other neural tube defects.[6] The U.S. Centers for Disease Control (CDC), the U.K. Department of Health, and many other public health authorities recommend that to prevent neural tube defects, all women thinking of having a baby should take a 400 microgram (0.4 milligram) folic acid supplement every day, in addition to natural dietary sources of folate.[7]

This should be considered a minimum, and some authorities recommend up to 800 micrograms for all women trying to conceive, or 4000 micrograms for women with a previous pregnancy affected by neural tube defects.[8]

Preventing birth defects is not the only reason to begin taking a prenatal multivitamin before pregnancy. Another benefit of starting early is that vitamins such as folic acid may help you conceive sooner and prevent miscarriage. The latest research clearly establishes that folate is important for every stage of fertility, from egg development to ovulation to fetal growth.[9]

Folate and Ovulation

Doctors have long suspected that vitamin deficiencies could play a role in ovulation problems in some women. This idea was supported by the results of the Nurses Health Study, which followed thousands of nurses over many years. The second round of the study followed a subgroup of more than 18 thousand women trying to conceive or who became pregnant, with no history of infertility, over 8 years.

When researchers at the Harvard School of Public Health analyzed the data from the Nurses Health Study, they found that the women who took a daily multivitamin were much less likely to have infertility due to ovulation problems. Taking a multivitamin just a few times per week was associated with a one-third lower chance of ovulatory infertility, and women who took a multivitamin every day had an even lower risk.[10] The researchers suggested that this was probably due to folic acid and other B vitamins.

The link between multivitamin use and fertility had actually been seen before in smaller studies in which researchers concluded that taking a multivitamin improves fertility.[11] These double-blind studies found higher pregnancy rates in women taking a multivitamin than women taking a placebo.

A diet higher in folate also increases progesterone levels and reduces the risk of ovulation disorders.[12] In one study, the third of women with the highest consumption of synthetic folate from fortified cereals had a 65% lower chance of ovulation disorders and had higher levels of progesterone at the time needed for optimal fertility.[13] Researchers now believe that having sufficient folate is critical for normal ovulation.[14]

Folate and Egg Quality

Folate also appears to improve egg quality and IVF success rates. Women who take folic acid supplements before IVF have also been found to have higher-quality eggs, and a higher proportion of mature eggs, than women not taking additional folate.[15] By measuring folate levels in the ovarian follicles of women undergoing IVF, Dutch researchers found that women with a twofold higher level of folic acid were three times more likely to become pregnant.[16]

A 2016 study by researchers at Oxford University also found that women with a mutation in the folate metabolism gene, MTHFR, were more likely to have chromosomally abnormal embryos and implantation failure, and were much less likely to become pregnant following IVF.[17] (These mutations have also long been associated with recurrent miscarriage.)

Mutations in the MTHFR gene are known to interfere with the processing of folic acid and folate to the biologically active form, methyl-folate, effectively reducing the level of active folate available. Approximately 40% of the population has a mutation in one copy of the gene, but this causes only a mild reduction in the ability to process folate (a 20-40% reduction in enzyme activity). Having a mutation in both copies of the gene has a much more significant impact, reducing the activity of the enzyme by up to 70%. These double mutations affect approximately 10% of the population. If you would like to know your genotype, your doctor can order a MTHFR blood test, or you can order DNA analysis yourself through 23andme then upload your data to the free website GeneticGenie.org.

Doctors typically recommended that women with an MTHFR mutation should take a much higher dose of folic acid (1000-4000 mcg) to make up for the reduced efficiency of processing folic acid to methyl-folate. It may, however, make more sense to choose a prenatal with folate already in the methyl-folate form, or to add a 400 mcg methyl-folate supplement to your existing prenatal. (Currently available methyl-folate prenatals are listed at www.itstartswiththeegg.com)

Studies have found that in women with MTHFR mutations, supplementing with methyl-folate is significantly more effective for raising blood folate levels than supplementing with folic acid.[18] Methyl-folate does, however, cause side effects in some people, such as muscle pain and mood changes, so it is not always the best option.

Rather than taking a very high dose of synthetic folic acid, or biologically active methyl-folate, a third option is to take a higher dose of actual folate. Before the MTHFR enzyme converts folate to methyl-folate, synthetic folic acid must first be converted to folate in the liver by the DHFR enzyme. Taking folate instead of folic acid skips this step and minimizes the concern of excess folic acid building up. While government bodies set upper limits of how much synthetic folic acid should be taken (1mg; or 4mg in the case of neural tube defects), no upper limit has been set for natural folate because, according to the NIH, "no adverse effects have been observed."[19]

Choosing natural folate over synthetic folic acid may in fact be wise even if you don't have a mutation in the MTHFR gene. The DHFR enzyme that converts synthetic folic acid to folate is not very efficient and varies significantly between different people. Given the critical importance of folate to ovulation, egg quality, and pregnancy rates, the last thing anyone needs is low folate levels due to poor conversion of synthetic folic acid. While most prenatals contain synthetic folic acid, it is possible to find brands that contain folate instead, or alternatively you can add a stand-alone supplement of natural folate to your existing prenatal. (See www.itstartswiththeegg.com for current brands).

Other Vitamins and Fertility

A typical prenatal multivitamin will contain several other vitamins that are also helpful for fertility, providing further reason to start taking a prenatal multivitamin even before pregnancy. For example, another vitamin that plays a role in egg quality is vitamin B12. Because this vitamin is typically obtained only from animal sources such as meat and dairy, vegans are usually deficient. In the same IVF study investigating the role of folate in women at a clinic in the Netherlands, researchers found that high levels of vitamin B12 are also associated with better embryo quality. This could be because vitamin B12, like folate, decreases homocysteine.[20]

Another specific vitamin that may improve fertility is vitamin B6. In 2007, Dr. Alayne Ronnenberg and scientists from the University of Illinois, Harvard Medical School, and Northwestern University published a study showing that women with low levels of vitamin B6 were less likely to become pregnant and more likely to miscarry.

All of this research indicates that taking a prenatal multivitamin that includes folic acid, vitamin B12, and vitamin B6 could make it much easier for you to become pregnant and reduce the risk of miscarriage and birth defects.

The minerals found in prenatal multivitamins may also be important during the time before pregnancy. For example, zinc, selenium, and iodine are necessary for proper thyroid function. This has implications for fertility because an underactive thyroid gland may suppress ovulation and raise the risk of miscarriage. Zinc and selenium are also involved in antioxidant defense systems and so likely play a role in egg quality, as discussed in the next chapter.

Choosing a Prenatal Multivitamin

There are so many prenatal multivitamin brands available that the choice can be bewildering, but just about any brand will have sufficient levels of the most important vitamins and minerals. Check for at least 2mg of B6, 6mcg of B12, 100mg of Iodine, 7mg of Zinc, and 50 mcg of Selenium. If you choose a prenatal that contains folic acid instead of folate or methylfolate, consider adding a stand-alone supplement of 400mcg of folate, or re-double your efforts to eat a folate-rich diet.

If you experience stomach problems from your prenatal multivitamins, try another brand and pay attention to the type of iron. You may not have the same problems with a supplement containing chelated iron. Many women who have nausea or other digestive issues from their prenatal multivitamin are able to take the supplements made by Rainbow Light or New Chapter Organics without any problems. Prenatal multivitamins are also less likely to upset your stomach if you take the tablet with a small meal or snack.

Recommended Dose

Take the dose recommended by your chosen brand of prenatal multivitamin, usually one tablet per day. Do not take more than the recommended dose, because a single dose may already have the daily limit of vitamin A, which can be toxic at high doses.

An Introduction to Other Supplements

The next several chapters will describe other specific supplements that you can take in addition to your prenatal multivitamin to improve egg quality. If you are going to add just one other supplement, make it Coenzyme Q10 (CoQ10 for short). As explained in the next chapter, the latest research suggests that taking CoQ10 increases egg and embryo quality by increasing the supply of cellular energy available to eggs. The safety of CoQ10 has been established in many large clinical studies, and it is likely that anyone trying to conceive can benefit from a CoQ10 supplement.

The subsequent chapters discuss additional supplements that may improve egg quality in women who are trying to conceive after 35 as well as women who have a history of infertility or previous miscarriages.

By way of general overview, Chapter 6 on CoQ10 and Chapter 7 on antioxidants and melatonin are generally applicable to anyone trying to conceive, although melatonin should not be taken unless you are trying to conceive by IVF. Chapter 8 on myo-inositol is more relevant to women with PCOS, irregular ovulation, or a history of miscarriage and insulin resistance. Chapter 9 on DHEA is relevant for women trying to conceive through IVF who have been diagnosed with diminished ovarian reserve or age-related infertility. Chapter 10 discusses why some so-called "fertility supplements," including pycnogenol, L-arginine, and royal jelly, are not recommended for anyone trying to conceive.

When to Start Taking Supplements and When to Stop

The specific timing depends on the supplement and your fertility concern, so discuss your plan with your doctor. However, the general strategy recommended by most fertility specialists is the following:

- Start taking a prenatal multivitamin as soon as possible and continue until after your baby is born and you stop nursing.

- If you are trying to conceive naturally, start other supplements such as Coenzyme Q10 or vitamin E as soon as possible and continue until you become pregnant.

- If you have PCOS, the above advice applies, but your doctor may also tell you to continue taking myo-inositol during your pregnancy to prevent gestational diabetes.

- If you are going through IVF, start all supplements at least two to three months before your egg retrieval if possible, and unless your doctor advises otherwise, stop all supplements when you begin stimulation medication (usually about a week or two before egg retrieval). Ask your doctor when to start taking your prenatal multivitamin again or whether you can continue taking it during the stimulation phase.

- If your IVF cycle is scheduled for less than three months away, there is likely still a benefit of starting supplements now. If nothing else, they can help you prepare for the next IVF cycle if your upcoming cycle is not successful.

- If you have a history of recurrent miscarriage, consider taking supplements for three months before trying to conceive again.

CHAPTER 6

The Power of Coenzyme Q10

"Energy and persistence conquer all things."
— *BENJAMIN FRANKLIN*

Recommended for:
Basic, Intermediate, and *Advanced Fertility Plans*

COENZYME Q10, OR CoQ10 for short, is a small molecule found in just about every cell in the body, including your eggs. Recent scientific research has revealed just how important this molecule is to preserving egg quality and fertility. Along with many other benefits, adding a CoQ10 supplement may have the potential to prevent or even reverse some of the decline in egg quality that comes with age.

Anyone trying to conceive can likely benefit from adding a CoQ10 supplement, but it is particularly helpful if you are in your mid-30s or older, or have fertility problems such as diminished ovarian reserve.

What Does CoQ10 Do?

CoQ10 has long been a favorite nutritional supplement of marathon runners and Olympic athletes,[1] and also a standard recommended supplement to prevent the muscle pain associated with cholesterol-lowering statin drugs. CoQ10 has also shown some initial promise in large clinical studies on a range of conditions that include congestive heart failure, Parkinson's, Huntington's, and Lou Gehrig's disease. But research has recently suggested yet another likely benefit of CoQ10 — improved egg quality.

How is it that one tiny molecule can do so much? It is probably because CoQ10 plays such an important role in making energy throughout the body — in muscles, the brain, and developing eggs. CoQ10 is in fact critical for energy production by the power plants inside our cells, mitochondria.

CoQ10 plays a direct role inside mitochondria by transferring electrons between other molecules. In other words, CoQ10 is a vital part of the "electron transport chain" that creates electrical energy (i.e., voltage) inside mitochondria. The mitochondria harness this electrical energy to make energy in the form of ATP. Cells then use ATP as the fuel to power just about every biological process.

CoQ10 is also an antioxidant that can recycle vitamin E and perform many other roles inside cells,[2] but it is the role this molecule plays in mitochondria that is most interesting for improving egg quality.

To understand how taking a CoQ10 supplement can improve egg quality, we first need to examine how poor egg quality relates to the supply of cellular energy and why this energy supply is compromised in the eggs of older women.

Energy for Eggs

As we age, mitochondria become damaged and are less efficient energy producers, much like an old, damaged power plant.[3] This decline in mitochondrial function is actually thought to play a key role in the aging process[4] and happens throughout the body, but particularly in eggs. Studies have specifically shown that in eggs from women over 40, structural damage to mitochondria is much more common.[5] Aging eggs also accumulate genetic damage in mitochondria,[6] and even the number of mitochondria decline in the follicle cells that surround each egg.[7]

As a result of all of this damage to mitochondria, and perhaps also as a result of declining CoQ10 levels with age, mitochondria in eggs from older women make less energy — that is, less ATP.[8] The inability to make enough ATP is a big problem for egg quality and is likely a major negative effect of aging on egg quality.[9]

But poorly functioning mitochondria are not just relevant to declining egg quality with age. There is also evidence of poor mitochondrial function in women with premature ovarian aging, including a condition known as primary ovarian insufficiency, and in women who have responded poorly to stimulation medication in IVF.[10]

A pioneer in this research, Dr. Jonathan Van Blerkom, first suggested in 1995 that there is a link between the ATP level in an egg and that egg's potential to mature properly and become a high-quality embryo.[11] This has since been confirmed by several researchers who have demonstrated that an egg's ability to produce a spike of ATP in the specific time and place needed for major developmental tasks is absolutely critical for proper egg development.[12]

Another piece of information confirming the theory that poorly functioning mitochondria are a big part of poor egg quality is the results of "cytoplasmic transfer." This experimental fertility procedure involved injecting a small percentage of the part of a young donor egg containing mitochondria into the eggs of older women with a history of infertility. This procedure "rescued" the poor quality eggs and significantly improved embryo development. Experts believe this occurred because the younger mitochondria were able to make up for the energy deficiency from older, poorly functioning mitochondria.[13]

Several children were born using this cytoplasmic transfer procedure before it was banned due to uncertainties about the health impacts of having two different kinds of mitochondria in the body. But the success of cytoplasmic transfer in helping women with poor egg quality become pregnant does indicate that if we can restore the function of mitochondria in eggs, we can significantly improve egg and embryo quality.

Having well-functioning mitochondria is now widely regarded as a hallmark of egg quality.[14] According to leading researchers in the field, the ability to make energy when needed is the single most important factor in determining the competence of eggs and embryos.[15] If an egg cannot produce energy when needed, it is likely to stop maturing or fail to fertilize.[16] Unsurprisingly, researchers have shown that artificially suppressing mitochondrial function during the time eggs are developing has a major negative effect on egg maturation and embryo viability.[17]

There is also a growing body of direct evidence that the ability of an egg to produce energy when needed is particularly important to being able to mature with the correct number of chromosomes. This is because the process of separating and ejecting chromosomes is very energy-intensive.[18] Scientists have actually seen the mitochondria cluster together and suddenly produce a burst of ATP at the precise time and place needed to form the structure that separates the chromosomes.[19]

If an egg does not have enough energy to neatly organize the chromosomes and separate the set of chromosomes to be pushed out, it may end up with an incorrect number of chromosome copies and will become an embryo with little chance of survival.

Just as we would expect, research has found that human embryos with poorly functioning mitochondria are more likely to have disrupted chromosomal processing machinery and chaotic chromosome distribution.[20] In addition, other researchers have shown that if you intentionally damage mitochondria in mouse eggs, the ATP level goes down, and the machinery that separates chromosomes disassembles and malfunctions.[21]

As discussed in earlier chapters, errors in the number of chromosome copies are the single greatest cause of failure of embryos to survive the first week, implantation failure, and early pregnancy loss. Chromosomal errors become much more common after the mid-30s and are also more common in people with a history of fertility problems or several early miscarriages. Suboptimal energy production by mitochondria may therefore directly contribute to infertility, failed IVF cycles, and early pregnancy loss by contributing to chromosome segregation errors in eggs.[22]

But energy supply is not just important for proper chromosomal processing — it also provides the fuel for the growing embryo. Problems with energy production in an egg can manifest later in embryo development because ATP is needed for all the work an embryo must do to grow to the blastocyst stage and successfully implant.[23] Dysfunctional mitochondria in eggs are thought to be especially problematic for early embryo survival.[24]

CoQ10 to Improve Egg Quality

Based on all the scientific knowledge about the importance of fully functioning mitochondria to egg and embryo quality, it stands to reason that anything we can do to boost mitochondrial function and help eggs produce more energy will improve egg quality and embryo viability. Research suggests that CoQ10 does just that.

As explained by Dr. Yaakov Bentov, a fertility specialist who has pioneered the use of CoQ10 to improve egg quality, "our thought is that it's not the egg that's different [in older women]; it's the ability of the egg to produce the kind of energy needed to complete all the processes that are involved with maturing and being fertilized. That's why we're recommending that women use all these supplements like co-enzyme Q10."[25]

The reason CoQ10 is such a widely used supplement and researchers are investigating it in a broad range of diseases is that it improves mitochondrial function.[26] Many studies have shown that adding CoQ10 to cells grown in the laboratory increases the production of ATP.[27] It has also been found to protect mitochondria from damage.[28]

If CoQ10 can do the same in eggs and increase the ATP supply needed to fuel egg development, this would be expected to prevent chromosomal errors and increase egg and embryo viability. While this has not yet been definitively proven in large clinical trials, scientific research indicates that CoQ10 can in fact improve egg quality, just as we would expect.

One of the earliest studies investigating CoQ10 and egg quality found that adding CoQ10 to cows' eggs growing in a laboratory more than doubled the proportion of eggs that grew to the five-day embryo stage. [29] It also increased the amount of ATP found within the embryos.

More recently, Dr. Bentov and his colleagues at the University of Toronto and Mount Sinai Hospital in Toronto have been leading the charge in investigating how CoQ10 can improve egg quality. They first found that the level of CoQ10 in cells surrounding mouse eggs declines with aging.[30] This discovery led the group to hypothesize that giving CoQ10 supplements to aging mice could perhaps slow or even reverse some of the effect of aging on egg quality and make the eggs from these older mice more like eggs from younger mice.

To investigate that question, the group gave CoQ10 to one-year-old mice (the equivalent of women in their late 40s) and found not only a significant increase in ATP production but, just as we would hope, an increase in the number of eggs ovulated after hormone stimulation.[31] The researchers concluded that "supplementing with mitochondrial nutrients such as

CoQ10 may lead to improvement in egg and embryo quality and pregnancy outcome."

As further evidence of the role of CoQ10 in egg quality, researchers in Italy have found higher levels of this molecule in ovarian follicles containing good-quality eggs. This was seen by analyzing the level of CoQ10 in the fluid of each ovarian follicle in 20 women undergoing IVF. The researchers saw higher CoQ10 levels in follicles containing mature eggs and eggs that gave rise to high-grade embryos.[32]

Researchers now believe that treating women with a CoQ10 supplement before an IVF cycle should increase mitochondrial activity and therefore increase egg numbers and quality.[33] There is, however, one important detail to keep in mind. Eggs take at least three to four months to develop, and CoQ10 takes several weeks or months to build up in tissues. For this reason, CoQ10 may be needed for as long as four to six months in advance of an IVF cycle to make a significant difference in the chance of success. This is all the more reason to start taking CoQ10 as soon as possible if you are trying to conceive.

Sources of CoQ10

CoQ10 is made in just about every cell in the body, so it is not technically a vitamin, and we do not need to obtain it from foods. But as we age, the body may not be able to make enough CoQ10 to keep up with the demands to make cellular energy.

Some foods do contain a substantial amount of CoQ10, such as sardines, meat, and poultry.[34] But studies have shown that increasing intake of these foods does not make much difference to CoQ10 levels in the body.[35] This is probably because even the foods with the highest content, such as sardines, really do not have that much. You would have to eat about three pounds of sardines every day to get the same amount of CoQ10 found in a typical supplement dose. So to improve your egg quality, a supplement form is really the only practical approach.

Supplementing CoQ10

Before we talk about how much CoQ10 to take and when, it is important to understand the two forms of this supplement to make sure you get the right one. These two forms are both naturally found in the body, and the only difference is a couple of electrons, but those electrons are important. The standard form in supplements is called **ubiquinone**. This form is not very soluble, so is not absorbed well. In the body, ubiquinone is converted (in chemistry-speak, "reduced") to the second form of CoQ10 to become an active antioxidant. This second form is called **ubiquinol**. More than 95% of the CoQ10 in circulation is in this reduced ubiquinol form,[36] and that is the form you want to buy because it is more easily absorbed.[37]

Even though it has been known for many years that the traditional supplement form, ubiquinone, is poorly absorbed, ubiquinol supplements were only introduced in 2006, because manufacturers had great difficulty finding a way to keep the active form stable in a supplement.

A Japanese company called Kaneka solved that problem, and most if not all ubiquinol in supplements is actually made by that company. This active ingredient is then formulated and packaged by different brands, most of which list KanekaQH on the back of the label. Some good-quality brands include Jarrow, GNC, and Life Extension.

If you just see a label that just says "CoQ10" without more information, you have to assume that it is the poorly absorbed ubiquinone because ubiquinol is more expensive to produce. Instead, you should look for the specific word "ubiquinol" on the label, or "active antioxidant form," or "reduced form." These supplements will be more expensive than traditional CoQ10 but may still offer better value because you can take a smaller dose and will absorb significantly more of the active ingredient.

Another option, although not as good as ubiquinol, is to choose a special formulation of ubiquinone that is designed to be more readily absorbed. Companies have gone to great lengths to figure out a way to make ubiquinone supplements work because they are much cheaper to produce. A variety of solutions have been developed to formulate ubiquinone in a way that increases absorption, such as suspending it in tiny droplets.[38]

Studies have shown that some of these high-tech formulations are absorbed significantly better than traditional ubiquinone supplements.[39] But there is likely no real advantage to ubiquinone other than lower cost, so ubiquinol is probably still a better choice.

Safety and Side Effects

Because CoQ10 holds promise in treating a range of diseases associated with impaired mitochondrial function, it has been studied extensively in large clinical trials. As part of these double-blind, placebo-controlled clinical studies, thousands of people have taken ubiquinone CoQ10 at high doses over many years and have been carefully observed. Researchers have reported no safety concerns, even at doses as high as 3000 mg/day. [40] At the time of writing, the only significant side effect reported in clinical studies is mild gastrointestinal symptoms in a small number of people.[41]

Although most large clinical studies have used ubiquinone, smaller studies have also shown that the more readily absorbed ubiquinol form is also safe.[42]

One other possible effect of CoQ10 to be aware of is that it has been reported to gradually improve blood sugar control in people with Type 2 diabetes,[43] although studies on this point have been inconsistent.[44] If you have diabetes, it is a good idea to discuss your plan to start taking CoQ10 with your doctor. Eventually your doctor may be able to reduce the dose of your diabetes medication.

Dose

Women enrolled in the clinical studies on CoQ10 and egg quality are given a daily dose of 600 mg of traditional CoQ10. This is equivalent to approximately 200–300 mg of ubiquinol.[45] The clinical studies were aimed at women aged 35–43 with previous IVF failures, so if you are not facing the same fertility hurdles, a smaller dose of 100 mg of ubiquinol is probably sufficient. You should talk to your doctor about what dose is right for you, but to give some examples of typical doses:

- Basic Fertility Plan: 100 mg ubiquinol (or 200 mg ubiquinone)

- Intermediate Fertility Plan: 200 mg ubiquinol (or 400 mg ubiquinone)

- Advanced Fertility Plan: 300 mg ubiquinol (or 600 mg ubiquinone)

CoQ10 is also absorbed better if you take it with a meal, and doctors recommend taking it with breakfast because it may boost energy too much at night and keep you awake.

It may be necessary to take CoQ10 for at least four months to have a significant effect on the chance of conceiving, but a shorter time is likely still beneficial.

Conclusion

Given everything we know about how CoQ10 increases energy production in mitochondria, how important this energy production is for egg and embryo development, how safe CoQ10 is, the fact that it is naturally found in the follicular fluid surrounding good-quality eggs, and the fact that it improves egg and embryo quality in animals and lab studies, the current evidence suggests that CoQ10 is worth taking even before we get crystal-clear proof from a large-scale human clinical study.

CHAPTER 7

Melatonin and
Other Antioxidants

*"All truth passes through three stages: First,
it is ridiculed; second, it is violently opposed;
third, it is accepted as self-evident."*
                    —ARTHUR SCHOPENHAUER

Recommended for:
Intermediate and *Advanced Fertility Plans*

ANTIOXIDANTS PLAY A vital role in egg quality by protecting against oxidative stress. Although ovarian follicles naturally contain a whole host of antioxidant vitamins and enzymes, these defenses are compromised in women with unexplained infertility, PCOS, and age-related infertility.

If you are young and have no fertility issues, a prenatal multivitamin and healthy diet will likely provide all the antioxidants you need. But if you are in your mid-30s or older, have

PCOS or unexplained infertility, or are preparing for IVF, you may need an additional antioxidant supplement to optimize egg quality.

What Are Antioxidants?

Antioxidants have long been known to play a role in fertility. The chemical name for vitamin E, tocopherol, was actually based on this important role, coming from the Greek word "tocos," meaning "childbirth," and "phero," meaning "to bring forth."[1] But vitamin E is just one of many antioxidants involved in fertility.

Some explanation of the terminology is useful to set the stage. The term "antioxidant" refers to a molecule that neutralizes reactive oxygen molecules. Reactive oxygen molecules are formed during normal metabolism and include "free radicals," which are particularly reactive because each oxygen molecule has an unpaired electron. The problem with reactive oxygen molecules, such as free radicals, is that when they react with other molecules, they cause oxidation.

The process of oxidization can be seen in everyday life, such as when metal rusts or silver tarnishes. Analogous chemical reactions occur inside cells. If not kept in check, oxidization can damage DNA, proteins, lipids, cell membranes, and mitochondria. But that is where antioxidants come in — they can be considered protectors against this chemical reaction of oxidation, analogous to using lemon juice to prevent an apple from turning brown.

Because of the potential of oxidants to cause cellular damage, each cell has an army of antioxidant defenses, including antioxidant enzymes produced with the specific purpose of neutralizing free radicals. Other important components of the antioxidant defense system are vitamins A, C, and E. Each of these antioxidants is found in developing eggs and has a role to play in preventing oxidative damage.

How Do Antioxidants Impact Egg Quality?

As we age, oxidative damage causes more and more problems for eggs.[2] This is in part due to a weakened antioxidant enzyme defense system in aging eggs; in eggs from older women, researchers have seen reduced production of antioxidant enzymes, which leaves more oxidizing molecules free to cause damage.[3] Unfortunately, eggs from older women also produce more oxidizing molecules to begin with because aging mitochondria "leak" electrons when they become damaged, which creates reactive oxidizing molecules.[4]

Mitochondria, those tiny power plants in every cell in the body, are actually a major source of reactive oxygen molecules and also a major victim.[5] Mitochondria are particularly sensitive to oxidative damage and release more oxidants when damaged, causing a vicious cycle resulting in more damage and more free radicals.[6]

All this oxidative damage to mitochondria reduces their ability to produce cellular energy in the form of ATP — energy that is critically important to egg development and embryo viability. Oxidative damage to mitochondria is now thought to be one of the major ways that aging impacts egg quality.

This oxidative damage is not limited to eggs from older women. Researchers have also found reduced antioxidant enzyme levels and higher levels of reactive oxygen molecules in women with unexplained infertility.[7] In one recent study, 70% of women with unexplained premature ovarian failure had elevated oxidation levels.[8] Even in eggs from young mice, oxidative stress decreases energy production and destabilizes chromosome processing.[9]

As a brief side note, an increased level of oxidative stress has also been seen in women with a history of PCOS, endometriosis, miscarriage, and preeclampsia.[10] With the exception of PCOS, it is not yet known what causes oxidative stress in these conditions, and the precise role of oxidative stress in endometriosis remains controversial.[11]

In women with PCOS, the condition often involves insulin resistance and high blood sugar. As a result of this high blood sugar, the body produces more reactive oxygen molecules, which increases oxidative stress.[12] (For the same reason, controlling blood sugar levels through diet, as discussed in Chapter 11, is particularly helpful in limiting oxidative stress at the source.)

Adding to this problem of increased oxidants in PCOS is the fact that PCOS is also associated with a decline in antioxidant activity.[13] As a result of these two hits, women with PCOS have higher levels of oxidation, which is thought to damage mitochondria and disrupt chromosome processing.[14] Poor egg quality as a result of oxidative stress is likely a major component of fertility problems in PCOS.[15]

The scientific research is also clear that eggs and embryos from older women, and women with fertility problems, have reduced antioxidant defense systems and are more sensitive to oxidative damage.[16] This oxidative damage is believed to damage mitochondria, compromising energy production and egg quality.[17]

Fortunately, antioxidants may be able to prevent some of this damage.[18] This idea is not without controversy, however, with one large review of prior studies concluding that there is no good quality evidence that antioxidant supplements increase live birth rates.[19] Yet since that review was published (in August 2013), more evidence has emerged that antioxidants do play an important role in fertility.[20]

For example, researchers have found that women with higher total antioxidant levels during IVF cycles have a greater chance of becoming pregnant.[21] Most recently, a large study of women undergoing fertility treatment at Boston IVF and Harvard Vanguard Medical Associates concluded that the use of antioxidant supplements was associated with a shorter time to pregnancy.[22] While there is still much more to investigate and many conflicting results so far, the balance of the current evidence suggests that having well-armed antioxidant defenses can protect eggs and improve fertility.

When it comes to determining which specific antioxidant supplements are most useful for fertility, initial research on vitamin C, vitamin E, alpha-lipoic acid, and N-acetyl cysteine is encouraging but not yet conclusive. For one antioxidant, however, a growing body of research consistently shows that it can significantly improve egg quality. That antioxidant is melatonin.

Melatonin

Melatonin is a hormone secreted at night by a small gland deep inside the brain, the pineal gland. You may know it as a natural sleep aid. Melatonin is used for this purpose because it regulates circadian rhythms, telling the body to go to sleep at night and wake up in the morning. It is so important in regulating sleep that exposure to bright light at night, which suppresses melatonin production in the brain, can compromise sleep quality and cause insomnia.

Melatonin is not just a sleep regulator, though — it is also involved in fertility. In some species, melatonin is involved in regulating seasonal fertility to ensure that lambs, calves, and other baby animals are born in spring.[23] Melatonin also plays a surprisingly important role in human fertility.

One clue that melatonin is important to human fertility is that particularly high levels of melatonin are found in the fluid of ovarian follicles.[24] Also, the amount of melatonin in the follicle fluid increases as the follicles grow. This was observed in women undergoing IVF, where higher levels of melatonin were found in larger, developed follicles than in small follicles.[25] Researchers have suggested that the increased level of melatonin as follicles grow has an important role in ovulation.[26]

Melatonin and Fertility

What exactly melatonin does in the ovaries is still not fully understood. Melatonin has traditionally been regarded as a hormonal messenger molecule that works by binding to specific receptors and thereby sending a message to cells. In other words, it was thought of as a molecule that merely communicates rather than having a direct biological effect. But in 1993, it was discovered that melatonin is also a powerful antioxidant that directly neutralizes free radicals.[27] This has since been confirmed by many different studies.[28] In some ways, melatonin is an even more powerful antioxidant than vitamin C and vitamin E.[29]

Unfortunately, melatonin levels decline with age,[30] and as a result, the ovaries lose this natural protector against oxidative stress. This could be one contributor to age-related infertility, but it is also a factor that can be changed. Scientists have recently discovered that taking a melatonin supplement can restore antioxidant defenses inside eggs and improve egg quality.

The story of melatonin and egg quality begins in the laboratory, where mouse eggs grown in the presence of the potent oxidant hydrogen peroxide were unable to develop properly. But when melatonin was added, the harmful effect of hydrogen peroxide was blocked.[31] This intriguing finding suggested that melatonin protected against oxidative stress, spurring further research.

Subsequent lab studies found that melatonin has this protective effect even without an added oxidizing agent. For example, in pig eggs cultured in the lab, those eggs grown with added melatonin were more likely to mature and had lower levels of reactive oxygen molecules.[32]

Melatonin has beneficial effects not just on eggs but also on embryos. Mouse embryos grown in a lab with melatonin showed an increased rate of forming blastocyst-stage embryos.[33] Melatonin also improved the development of pig and cow embryos,[34] and researchers determined that this was at least in part due to antioxidant activity.

All these studies led doctors to believe that melatonin may also improve egg and embryo quality in women undergoing IVF. And so the human clinical trials began. In one of the first studies giving melatonin to women undergoing IVF, researchers found that melatonin lowered levels of oxidative stress and cellular oxidative damage in ovarian follicles — a very promising discovery.[35]

Researchers then found that melatonin not only reduces oxidative damage but also improves egg and embryo quality. In a study led by Dr. Hiroshi Tamura, nine women were given melatonin from the beginning of an IVF cycle, and their egg quality was compared to each woman's previous cycle. After treatment with melatonin, there was a dramatic improvement, with an average of 65% of their eggs giving rise to good-quality embryos, compared to just 27% in the previous cycle.[36]

The next step was to investigate the impact of melatonin on the actual pregnancy rate in IVF to see if melatonin really increased the chance of becoming pregnant. To that end, Dr. Tamura and a group of doctors in Japan performed a trailblazing clinical study involving 115 women who had a previous failed IVF cycle and a low fertilization rate.[37] Before undertaking another IVF cycle, half the women were given melatonin. These women went on to have a fertilization rate much higher than the previous cycle, and nearly 20% of the melatonin-treated women became pregnant.

By contrast, the women not given melatonin had the same low fertilization rate as their previous cycle, and only 10% of these women became pregnant. These results demonstrated that melatonin improved the fertilization rate and nearly doubled the chance of becoming pregnant through IVF.

Dr. Tamura noted: "Our study represents the first clinical application of melatonin treatment for infertility patients. This work needs to be confirmed, but we believe that melatonin treatment is likely to become a significant option for improving oocyte quality in women who cannot become pregnant because of poor oocyte quality."[38]

In a similar study, this time in Italy, doctors found that a daily melatonin supplement before IVF increased the proportion of mature versus immature eggs and led to a higher number of top-quality embryos.[39]

These studies together show that melatonin can be particularly beneficial for women undergoing IVF who have had failed IVF cycles due to poor egg quality.

Unfortunately, it is probably not a good idea to take a melatonin supplement if you are trying to conceive naturally because it appears that melatonin may have a direct role in regulating the production of hormones that control the ovulation cycle.[40] A melatonin supplement may therefore disrupt the natural hormone balance and interfere with ovulation.

This is not such a concern in the context of IVF because large doses of hormones are given to artificially regulate the cycle, and ovulation does not need to be carefully orchestrated by natural hormone levels. For women about to go through an IVF cycle, melatonin is so beneficial for egg quality that any minor effects on hormones are seen as irrelevant. For women trying to conceive naturally, the reverse is probably true, and disrupting ovulation may be too high a price to pay for improved egg quality.

If you are trying to conceive without IVF, one possible approach to getting some of melatonin's benefits without the risk of disrupting ovulation is to naturally restore normal melatonin levels through exposure to light. For example, taking the opportunity to go for a walk outside early in the day may help because more than an hour or two of bright sunlight during the day increases melatonin levels at night.[41] By contrast, bright light at night can artificially suppress melatonin levels, so it is wise to dim the lights and avoid screen time in the hour or two before bed.

Some foods also contain small amounts of melatonin, including tart cherries. The easiest way to take advantage of this natural melatonin source is to drink tart cherry juice at night. The highest concentration is found in the Montmorency variety of tart cherries, the juice of which can be found online. Other foods that contain small amounts of melatonin include barley and walnuts. But if you are preparing for an IVF cycle, the easiest way to obtain enough melatonin to maximize egg quality is through a supplement.

Adding a Melatonin Supplement

Fertility clinics that stay abreast of scientific research now routinely recommend melatonin supplements for women preparing for IVF cycles, particularly when poor egg quality is a concern.

The dose of melatonin used in the clinical studies on egg quality in IVF is a 3 mg tablet shortly before bed, starting at the beginning of the IVF cycle – typically the day when a GnRH antagonist such as Lupron is started. Melatonin supplements may cause daytime drowsiness, dizziness, and irritability, and may worsen depression.[42] If side effects bother you, switching to a smaller dose is likely to help.

Other Fertility-Boosting Antioxidants

If you are trying to conceive without IVF and therefore melatonin is not the right supplement for you, alternative antioxidant supplements may have similar benefits. Although these other antioxidants are not supported by the same clear evidence demonstrating their ability to improve egg quality, it is worth considering adding one of them to your supplement regimen. These other antioxidants can also be used in conjunction with melatonin if you are preparing for IVF and are particularly concerned about your egg quality.

Vitamin E

Vitamin E is a fat-soluble antioxidant found in nuts, seeds, and oil. Preliminary research in animals and humans now suggests that vitamin E could have a beneficial effect on egg quality.[43] One of the most interesting examples is a human study that compared the ability of vitamin E and melatonin to reduce free radical damage in ovarian follicles. The researchers found that both supplements were effective, although a 200-times higher dose of vitamin E was required for the same level of protection against free radicals.[44] That is, 600 mg of vitamin E had a similar effect to 3 mg of melatonin.

This study used a high dose of vitamin E — about double the recommended maximum daily dose. To explain this in practical terms, vitamin E supplements are often labeled with "IU" for International Units, and 600 mg is equivalent to 900 IU. A typical prenatal multivitamin will contain 30–60 IU, while a typical vitamin E supplement will contain 400 IU.

Although vitamin E is generally regarded as very safe, the European Food Safety Authority has indicated that adults should not take more than 300 mg daily, [45] which is equivalent to 450 IU. [46]

The Colorado Center for Reproductive Medicine (CCRM), arguably the top IVF clinic in the U.S., recommends that women preparing for IVF take 200 IU of vitamin E because "studies [suggest] that 400 IU may not be as good for overall health."[47] CCRM also warns that vitamin E should not be used by people who are taking aspirin, because it adds to the anti-clotting effect of aspirin.

While a vitamin E supplement alone may not be enough to dramatically improve egg quality, every small incremental improvement in egg quality helps.

A study published in 2014 by Dr. Elizabeth Ruder and other researchers at the University of Pittsburgh, Emory University, and Dartmouth Medical Center adds further support to the view that vitamin E supplements are particularly useful for women with unexplained infertility.[48] The study involved over 400 women with unexplained infertility who were trying to conceive through IUI and IVF. The researchers found that in the women who were over age 35, greater intake of vitamin E through supplements was linked to a shorter time to pregnancy.

Although further research is needed, experts now believe that vitamin E may compensate for some of the decline in antioxidant levels that naturally occurs as women age.[49] If you decide to take a vitamin E supplement in addition to the small amount of vitamin E in your prenatal multivitamin, it is best to err on the side of caution and look for one that contains no more than 200 IU.

Vitamin C

Vitamin C is a water-soluble antioxidant naturally found in large amounts in ovarian follicles.[50] In older mice, both vitamins C and E were found to prevent at least some of the age-related decline in ovarian function.[51] A vitamin C derivative also improved the quality of pig embryos in a lab study. In human studies, however, there is still limited evidence that taking additional vitamin C improves female fertility.

One of the few studies to date showing positive results from the use of vitamin C supplements is the same 2014 study described above in the context of vitamin E. In addition to investigating the value of vitamin E supplements, the study also explored whether vitamin C supplements were helpful to women with unexplained infertility.

The researchers found that at least for women of a healthy weight and women under the age of 35, increased vitamin C intake from supplements was associated with a shorter time to pregnancy.[52] This does not mean that vitamin C is thought to be less helpful to older or overweight women, but rather the effect was not seen in the study because the dose may have been too low for these groups. The researchers explained that in the overweight women, and most women in the older age bracket, their vitamin C intake was likely not sufficient to make up for their already high levels of oxidation.

If you choose to add a vitamin C supplement, CCRM recommends a dose of 500 mg.[53]

Alpha-Lipoic Acid

Alpha-lipoic acid is another supplement that has well-established antioxidant properties and may therefore benefit egg quality.[54] It is naturally produced in the body and has the rare ability to act as both a water-soluble and fat-soluble antioxidant.[55] By contrast, vitamin C is water soluble and Vitamin E is fat soluble, so those antioxidants have more limited reach.

Alpha-lipoic acid is also a promising supplement because it is found naturally in mitochondria, where it assists in energy production.[56] Animal studies have found that alpha-lipoic acid can protect mitochondria from the effects of aging.[57] When people take alpha-lipoic acid supplements, the total antioxidant level in the bloodstream increases significantly, and there is an increase in the activity of antioxidant enzymes.[58]

There is also some evidence that alpha-lipoic acid improves fertility. For example, laboratory studies have found that this antioxidant can improve egg maturation and embryo viability.[59]

The fertility specialists in Toronto who led the groundbreaking research into CoQ10 also investigated the ability of alpha-lipoic acid to improve egg numbers and quality. They gave mice supplements of either CoQ10 or alpha-lipoic acid to test the hypothesis that both compounds are antioxidants that should improve mitochondrial function and thereby improve egg quality. The researchers thought that both CoQ10 and alpha-lipoic acid would be particularly helpful because they are not just antioxidants but are also directly involved in the activity of mitochondria.[60]

While this research found that CoQ10 improved egg numbers and quality, alpha-lipoic acid did not seem to have the same benefit.[61] Nevertheless, in a paper published in 2013, three years after these disappointing results, the same researchers maintained that supplementing with mitochondrial nutrients such as alpha-lipoic acid may improve egg and embryo quality and may lead to a healthy pregnancy for older women.[62]

There is also some direct evidence that alpha-lipoic acid may specifically improve fertility in women with PCOS, with one study finding that women taking 600 mg twice a day for 16 weeks had improved insulin sensitivity and began ovulating normally.[63]

Therefore, even though the general ability of alpha-lipoic acid to improve egg quality has not yet been proven in large clinical studies, experts in this area are not giving up hope that alpha-lipoic acid may help, and not just in the context of PCOS. There is a solid theoretical reason why it should improve egg quality, and it is regarded as very safe,[64] so it may be worth trying in addition to more proven supplements such as CoQ10 and melatonin.

Safety and Side Effects of Alpha-Lipoic Acid

In clinical trials of alpha-lipoic acid, no significant side effects have been reported. The most common side effect is nausea, but even this is rare at doses of 600 mg per day. [65]

It has been suggested that alpha-lipoic acid may lower thyroid hormones,[66] so if you have thyroid problems, you should not take this supplement before discussing it with your doctor. Alpha-lipoic acid may also improve blood sugar levels in diabetics,[67] so if you have diabetes you should be carefully monitored when you start taking this supplement. Ultimately, your doctor may be able to decrease the dose of your diabetes medication.

Dosage and Form of Alpha-Lipoic Acid

Because there has been very little research on the effectiveness of alpha-lipoic acid for improved egg quality, it is difficult to determine the appropriate dose. The best we can do is to choose the dose typically used in clinical trials and shown to be effective for other conditions, such as diabetic nerve pain. [68] This dose is 600 mg per day (although the study showing a benefit in PCOS gave women double this dose — 600 mg, twice per day). If you are unsure about whether you want to take this supplement, you could instead try a lower dose of 100 mg per day, which is another standard dosage found in alpha-lipoic acid supplements.

Before choosing an alpha-lipoic acid supplement, it is important to know what form to look for. When alpha-lipoic acid is synthesized in the body, it is made in one specific form, called R-alpha-lipoic acid.[69] When it is made in the lab, however, one of the chemical groups can be flipped so that the molecule as a whole is a mirror image of R-alpha-lipoic acid (the same way your left hand is a mirror image of your right hand).

Many alpha-lipoic acid supplements are a mixture of these two forms, having left-handed and right-handed molecules. If you can find a supplement specifically labeled as "r-alpha-lipoic acid," or "R-lipoic acid" for short, it is a better choice because this is the natural form made in the body, is more readily absorbed, and is likely to be more effective.[70]

Alpha-lipoic acid may also be better absorbed on an empty stomach, so to get the most from this supplement, you should take it 30 minutes before or 2 hours after eating. [71]

N-Acetyl Cysteine

Another antioxidant that may benefit egg quality and fertility is called N-acetyl cysteine. This amino acid derivative acts as an antioxidant and also boosts the activity of another critical antioxidant inside cells, called glutathione.[72] It is commonly used as an antidote to poisoning from overdose of acetaminophen (also known as Tylenol or paracetamol).[73]

Most research into N-acetyl cysteine and fertility has focused on PCOS, finding that N-acetyl cysteine boosts ovulation and increases the chance of pregnancy when taken by women with PCOS in conjunction with an ovulation-inducing drug such as Clomid.

In one clinical trial, women with PCOS took N-acetyl

cysteine and Clomid for 5 days per cycle for 12 cycles. The pregnancy rates increased from 57% for women taking the placebo to 77% for women taking N-acetyl cysteine. The group taking N-acetyl cysteine also had improved ovulation rates and much lower miscarriage rates.[74]

Another similar clinical trial saw even more striking results. Women with PCOS who on average had suffered from infertility for more than 4 years took N-acetyl cysteine and the ovulation-stimulating drug Clomid for 5 days. After treatment, 45% of the women taking N-acetyl cysteine ovulated, compared to 28% in the placebo group. In addition, 21% of the women taking N-acetyl cysteine became pregnant, compared to 9% of women taking the placebo.

The authors hypothesized that N-acetyl cysteine may improve ovulation in PCOS by improving insulin response.[75] Other researchers have seen that N-acetyl cysteine does indeed reduce insulin and testosterone levels in PCOS.[76]

But N-acetyl cysteine is also an antioxidant, and for this reason researchers believe it may also improve egg quality and fertility in women without PCOS. Specifically, by acting as an antioxidant, it may counteract the effect of aging on egg quality.

So far, the evidence supporting this idea comes only from very recent studies on animals, but this research is quite promising. For example, in 2012 a group of researchers from Nankai University in China, the University of Ottawa, and New York University Langone Medical Center published the results of a study in which mice were given N-acetyl cysteine for two months or one year.[77] The researchers then determined the number and quality of the mice's eggs and embryos. They found that even short-term treatment improved the number and quality of fertilized eggs and also improved embryo development. Long-term use in mice appeared to prevent the usual age-related decline in fertility.

The authors of this study suggested that the beneficial effect on egg and embryo quality was due to the antioxidant properties of N-acetyl cysteine and that by reducing oxidative stress in the ovaries, this supplement could prevent or delay ovarian aging. In fact, earlier research by some of the same researchers indicated that N-acetyl cysteine reduces oxidative stress, reduces chromosomal damage, reduces chromosomal instability, and improves egg and embryo development.[78]

In separate research also published in 2012, immature eggs were isolated from pig ovaries and grown in the lab with or without N-acetyl cysteine.[79] The researchers saw a significant decrease in the percentage of eggs with fragmented DNA and an increase in the percentage of embryos reaching the blastocyst stage when eggs were treated with N-acetyl cysteine. There was also an improvement in egg and embryo development.

Although not yet confirmed by human studies, we may be on the cusp of seeing significant benefit for egg and embryo quality in humans as well, and N-acetyl cysteine may become a more commonly recommended supplement for women preparing for IVF.

Based on current research, all we know is that N-acetyl cysteine seems to be very helpful in improving fertility in women with PCOS, but since it is a powerful antioxidant, it may improve egg and embryo quality in other women, too.

Another intriguing trend supported by research on N-acetyl cysteine is that it could decrease miscarriage risk. A group of women with unexplained recurrent miscarriage were given 600 mg per day along with folic acid, and the pregnancy outcomes compared to women taking folic acid alone. The combination of N-acetyl cysteine and folic acid was associated with a very dramatic decrease in the chance of miscarriage. Women taking N-acetyl cysteine were twice as likely to take a baby home as women not taking N-acetyl cysteine.[80]

Other studies have also shown that N-acetyl cysteine decreases the miscarriage rate by 60% in women with PCOS.[81] It appears that this benefit is not limited to women with PCOS, so you may want to consider taking an N-acetyl cysteine supplement if you have suffered multiple unexplained miscarriages.

Safety and Side Effects of N-Acetyl Cysteine

N-acetyl cysteine is widely used by doctors for a variety of conditions,[82] but the safety record of this supplement is not entirely reassuring. For example, serious allergic reactions have occurred after the use of N-acetyl cysteine to treat painkiller overdose.[83] An allergic reaction to N-acetyl cysteine may be particularly dangerous if you are asthmatic.[84] If you decide to take N-acetyl cysteine, you should do so under a doctor's supervision and find out more about the safety risks.

Dosage of N-Acetyl Cysteine

The dose used to treat women with PCOS in clinical trials is 1.2 g per day, but this use was very short-term. The women were only given N-acetyl cysteine for five days, corresponding with the five-day dose of Clomid.[85] In the study on recurrent miscarriage, the dose was 600 mg per day.

Conclusion

Many experts believe that oxidative stress is a major mechanism underlying ovarian aging.[86] To prevent oxidative damage to eggs, reactive oxygen molecules (such as free radicals) must be continuously kept in check by the eggs' natural antioxidants. But in women with age-related infertility, PCOS, or unexplained infertility, this natural antioxidant defense system may be compromised, creating a need for further antioxidants.

Melatonin is one of the most effective antioxidants for improving egg quality but may potentially disrupt ovulation in women trying to conceive naturally. Melatonin is therefore most useful if you are trying to conceive through IVF, while vitamin E, vitamin C, or alpha-lipoic acid is a better option if you are trying to conceive naturally.

CHAPTER 8

Restoring Ovulation with Myo-Inositol

*"Sometimes the questions are complicated
and the answers are simple."*

— DR. SEUSS

Recommended for:
Intermediate and *Advanced Fertility Plans*

MYO-INOSITOL IS PARTICULARLY helpful for restoring ovulation and improving egg quality in women with PCOS or insulin resistance. It may also reduce the miscarriage risk associated with insulin resistance.

Not recommended for:

Many studies have shown that myo-inositol is very safe, with few or no side effects. Myo-inositol should, however, be used with caution if you have schizophrenia or bipolar disorder because there is a theoretical risk of exacerbating manic episodes.[1]

Why Myo-Inositol?

Myo-inositol has recently become a widely recommended fertility supplement, yet the story of myo-inositol's role in egg quality began more than 10 years ago. In 2002, Dr. Tony Chiu and a group of researchers in Hong Kong published the results of the first study to directly link this B vitamin to egg and embryo quality.[2] They found the link by tracking the levels of myo-inositol inside each ovarian follicle in 53 women undergoing IVF and then comparing the amount of myo-inositol in each follicle to the quality of the egg inside and whether it later fertilized.

The results were unambiguous. Higher levels of myo-inositol were found in ovarian follicles containing mature eggs that later successfully fertilized than in follicles containing immature eggs that failed to fertilize. This same study also uncovered a relationship between the concentration of myo-inositol in the ovarian follicles and embryo quality. A higher amount of myo-inositol was found in follicles containing eggs that developed into good-quality embryos.

Dr. Chiu was inspired to investigate the levels of myo-inositol in ovarian follicles by much earlier research showing that this compound is a precursor to important signaling molecules called inositol phospholipids.[3] These signaling molecules communicate messages and thereby regulate a wide range of biological activities inside cells, including in developing eggs.

The new link between higher levels of myo-inositol

and higher-quality eggs raised an intriguing possibility to researchers: Perhaps adding extra myo-inositol in the form of a supplement could improve egg quality and fertility. It took more than five years to test that hypothesis, and studies proved that the answer wasn't quite so simple. It turns out that myo-inositol supplements only have a clear benefit in women with PCOS or insulin resistance.

Myo-Inositol and PCOS

To understand why myo-inositol is beneficial in PCOS, we need to go back to the underlying cause of the hormonal imbalances in this condition. Doctors have known for more than 30 years that PCOS is associated with high insulin levels, even in women of a healthy weight.[4] High insulin levels appear to have a direct role in causing infertility in PCOS by increasing levels of hormones such as testosterone in the ovaries.[5]

Based on this understanding, PCOS has been treated with various drugs that make the body more responsive to insulin. These drugs aim to make cells more sensitive to insulin's message to take up glucose from the bloodstream, thereby better controlling blood glucose levels and lowering insulin levels. One example is metformin, which has been widely studied for improving blood sugar control in PCOS and diabetes.[6]

The theory of using metformin to improve fertility in PCOS is that by returning insulin levels to normal, we could also rebalance reproductive hormones and restore ovulation. Metformin, however, has some significant side effects, such as nausea and vomiting,[7] and it is not clear how well it works.

Against this background, scientists began looking for

alternatives for improving insulin function in women with PCOS, with the goal of ultimately improving fertility. This is where the story returns to myo-inositol. It was already known that some molecules in the inositol family are involved in insulin function and sugar metabolism. It was also known that myo-inositol may be depleted in PCOS. The final piece of the puzzle was Dr. Chiu's experiments showing higher levels of myo-inositol in follicles associated with good-quality eggs.

Putting all this together led doctors to suspect that perhaps myo-inositol could improve insulin activity, ovulation, and egg quality in women with PCOS. And they were right.

Many studies have now consistently shown that taking a myo-inositol supplement is beneficial in women with PCOS. In one of the first studies, published in 2007, 25 women with PCOS took a myo-inositol supplement for six months. Before the study began, all these women had experienced at least 1 year of infertility and less than 6 menstrual cycles per year, and it had been determined that the most likely cause of their infertility was ovulation dysfunction. Over the course of the 6 months taking myo-inositol, 72% of these women began ovulating normally again.[8] More than half of these women then became pregnant.

Similar results were reached in several later studies, [9] including a study in which both doctor and patient were blind as to whether a particular patient was assigned to myo-inositol or a placebo, minimizing the possibility of bias and the placebo effect. [10] The results were stark: In women receiving myo-inositol, nearly 70% ovulated compared to just 21% ovulating after taking the placebo.

All these studies showing restored ovulation and improved

chances of conceiving naturally are just one part of the story. At a more granular level, IVF cycles have also allowed doctors to directly observe the positive impact of myo-inositol on egg and embryo quality in women with PCOS.

In the first IVF study showing this positive impact, women were given myo-inositol starting on the day of the IVF medications. Myo-inositol was found to increase the proportion of mature eggs retrieved and decrease the number of immature and degenerated eggs, compared to women not receiving myo-inositol.[11] In addition, fewer cycles were canceled because of concern about overstimulating the ovaries.

When the myo-inositol supplement was started earlier, it had an even greater impact on IVF outcomes in women with PCOS.[12] In a double-blind trial, doctors gave women 2 grams of myo-inositol plus folic acid twice a day for three months and gave a second group folic acid alone. When the women underwent IVF, those who had been taking myo-inositol had more mature follicles, more eggs retrieved, and fewer immature eggs retrieved compared to women taking folic acid alone. Interestingly, this study also found a much higher proportion of top-quality embryos in women taking myo-inositol: 68% versus 29% in the women taking only folic acid.

In short, myo-inositol seems to improve egg development and embryo quality in women with PCOS, along with lowering insulin and improving blood sugar control. And it is not just women with poor insulin sensitivity who can benefit. A study conducted in Italy and published in 2011 found that even in PCOS patients having a normal insulin response, myo-inositol treatment improved egg and embryo quality during IVF.[13]

How Does Myo-Inositol Improve Egg Quality in PCOS?

Myo-inositol may improve egg quality in women with PCOS by acting as a precursor to specific signaling molecules that are critical to egg development.[14] Although the mechanism is not fully understood, researchers believe that a defect in the processing of molecules in the inositol family may contribute to insulin resistance in PCOS.[15] A myo-inositol supplement may circumvent this problem and allow normal signaling inside developing eggs.[16]

PCOS and Gestational Diabetes

If you have PCOS, taking a myo-inositol supplement while trying to conceive could have another added benefit: reducing your risk of gestational diabetes. This condition, which involves high blood sugar levels during pregnancy, is much more common in women with PCOS.

In 2012, researchers found that women with PCOS taking a myo-inositol supplement during their pregnancy had a much lower risk of gestational diabetes: just 17% compared to 54% in women not taking the supplement.[17] Thus myo-inositol may provide an effective way to keep blood sugar under control during pregnancy and prevent gestational diabetes. If you have PCOS, you should therefore ask your doctor whether to continue taking myo-inositol during pregnancy.

What if You Don't Have PCOS?

Unfortunately, when it comes to improving fertility in women without PCOS or insulin resistance, it appears that myo-inositol is not very helpful. We would expect myo-inositol to have a general benefit for egg quality based on Dr. Chiu's 2002 study showing a link between high levels of myo-inositol in follicles and good-quality eggs, but this has not led to the results we would expect in human studies.

In a recent study in Italy in which doctors gave myo-inositol to women without PCOS for three months before an IVF cycle, the results were unimpressive. Myo-inositol actually seemed to reduce the number of mature eggs and embryos. [18] While the implantation rate and pregnancy rates were slightly higher in the myo-inositol group compared to the group given a placebo, the study was too small to test whether this difference was real or occurred by chance.

As the authors of the study pointed out, reducing the number of eggs maturing in an IVF cycle is not all bad — it could mean that myo-inositol will reduce the risk of ovarian hyperstimulation, which is an occasional outcome of IVF cycles in which too many follicles mature at the same time, causing dangerous complications.

Yet the clear implication of the current research is that myo-inositol has much more value in women with PCOS than other forms of infertility. Myo-inositol may, however, be worth considering if you have not been diagnosed with PCOS but either have insulin resistance or are not ovulating regularly and your doctor cannot determine the cause. It may be that you share some of the underlying hormonal imbalances common to PCOS and could benefit from a myo-inositol supplement to restore normal ovulation.

Myo-Inositol and Miscarriage

Myo-inositol may also have a role to play in preventing miscarriage in women with recurrent pregnancy loss. Studies have found a much higher rate of insulin resistance in women with a history of multiple miscarriages.[19] In one study, insulin resistance was two to three times more common in this group.[20] Insulin resistance is similarly thought to increase the risk of miscarriage in women with PCOS.[21]

In theory, if insulin resistance contributes to the risk of miscarriage, a supplement that reverses insulin resistance, such as myo-inositol, could be beneficial. But this use of myo-inositol would be speculative because miscarriage can have many other causes unrelated to insulin levels. Nevertheless, given the safety of myo-inositol, you may want to consider adding it to your supplement list if you have lost multiple pregnancies and want to try everything you can to reduce your risk.

Safety, Side Effects, and Dose

Myo-inositol has been described as very safe, with only high doses of 12 g per day causing mild gastrointestinal symptoms such as nausea.[22] The typical recommended dose, shown to be effective in clinical studies, is 4 g per day, divided into two doses: half in the morning and half at night.

What About D-Chiro Inositol?

A similar-sounding and related compound, D-chiro inositol, is often used by women with PCOS in the hope of improving their fertility, but it may have just the opposite effect: reducing the number and quality of eggs.[23] This negative effect is unfortunately not widely known. The early studies showing a possible benefit of D-chiro inositol have overshadowed the more recent studies showing that the supplement simply does not work or may do more harm than good.[24] As just one example of the recent research raising a red flag for this supplement, an Italian study published in 2012 found that women with PCOS who were given D-chiro inositol rather than a placebo had fewer eggs and fewer good-quality embryos. [25]

Researchers are beginning to understand why D-chiro inositol is unhelpful in PCOS. It appears that PCOS may involve overactive conversion of myo-inositol into D-chiro inositol, depleting normal levels of myo-inositol.[26] This could in turn cause poor egg quality, which would explain why myo-inositol could improve egg quality, while D-chiro inositol could simply make the problem worse.

Conclusion

Myo-inositol is now routinely recommended for women with PCOS because it appears to restore normal ovulation, improve egg quality, and prevent gestational diabetes. If you have PCOS, taking a daily myo-inositol supplement for several weeks or months could be the missing link that allows you to become pregnant naturally. Myo-inositol may also improve fertility in women who do not ovulate or who have insulin resistance. There is a possibility that myo-inositol could also reduce miscarriage risk by lowering insulin levels, but further research is needed.

CHAPTER 9

DHEA for Diminished Ovarian Reserve

"Don't be discouraged. It's often the last key
in the bunch that opens the lock."

— UNKNOWN

Recommended for: *Advanced Plan*

DHEA IS NOW widely recommended by IVF clinics for improving egg quality and egg numbers in women with diminished ovarian reserve or age-related infertility who are preparing for IVF.[1]

Not recommended for:

Even though DHEA is sold over the counter as a nutritional supplement, it is actually a hormone so you should talk to your fertility specialist before taking it. You should not take DHEA if you have PCOS or certain cancers.

An Introduction to DHEA

The story of DHEA started with one woman, a determined patient at an IVF clinic in New York who was over 40 and searching for anything that could improve her odds. In her own research, she uncovered a scientific article about DHEA improving egg numbers in IVF and started taking the supplement. The results were so astounding that her clinic quickly became pioneers in the use of DHEA to improve IVF outcomes. Several years later, DHEA is now routinely recommended for certain IVF patients to increase the number and quality of eggs and embryos. According to Dr. Norbert Gleicher, a leading fertility specialist, "DHEA is in the process of revolutionizing infertility care for older women and for younger women with premature aging ovaries."[2]

DHEA has, however, been plagued by controversy for many years, and even now IVF clinics are divided on its value. The research showing the benefits of DHEA has been hailed by some experts as a major breakthrough and criticized by others for improper study design. There are still many unknowns, but the weight of the evidence so far suggests that there is very good reason for women with diminished ovarian reserve to take DHEA for three months before an IVF cycle.

What Is DHEA?

DHEA, which stands for dehydroepiandrosterone, is a hormone precursor produced by the adrenals and ovaries as an intermediate step in the production of estrogen and testosterone. Because it is a precursor to estrogen and testosterone, when taken as a supplement it can increase the level of these hormones in the ovaries.[3]

Levels of DHEA usually decline with age,[4] and as a result some have touted its use as an anti-aging supplement and as a treatment to relieve menopause symptoms. DHEA has also been used by athletes as a performance-enhancing substitute for anabolic steroids.[5] The research described in this chapter suggests that DHEA may also help some IVF patients increase the number and quality of eggs retrieved and thereby increase the chance of becoming pregnant.

The Discovery of DHEA Boosting Fertility

The pioneers in the use of DHEA to increase fertility are the reproductive endocrinologists at the Center for Human Reproduction (CHR), a large IVF clinic in New York with a surprisingly high success rate in older patients having low ovarian reserve. Their work on DHEA began with a single patient, a 43-year-old woman scouring the medical literature for anything that could help improve her egg numbers.

In her first IVF cycle, before taking DHEA, she produced just a single egg and embryo, and her doctors discouraged further attempts at IVF using her own eggs. Determined to have a child with her own eggs, she began her own search of the scientific literature for anything that could help.

During this research, she stumbled upon a publication from researchers at Baylor University suggesting a possible benefit of DHEA in IVF cycles.[6] The Baylor study described an increase in egg numbers in five women taking DHEA for two months, but received very little attention until it was rediscovered and put to the test several years later by this individual patient in New York.

After reading the Baylor paper, she began taking DHEA

supplements, unbeknownst to her doctors. In her second IVF cycle, she produced three eggs and embryos.

Amazingly, as she continued taking DHEA, her egg and embryo numbers progressively increased.[7] She explains, "I was beginning to realize I was onto something."[8] Her doctors report being astonished because at her age she should have been getting worse, not better.[9] She ultimately produced 16 embryos in her ninth IVF cycle.[10]

This continuous improvement in egg numbers suggested that the beneficial effects of DHEA were cumulative. It is now understood that this longer-term effect is because DHEA acts on very early-stage follicles that are several months away from ovulation.

By 2011, just six years after the first extraordinary results with DHEA, a substantial number of IVF clinics worldwide began recommending DHEA supplements for women with diminished ovarian reserve.[11] This recommendation is in line with a series of studies suggesting that DHEA really does improve IVF outcomes in women who are otherwise unlikely to have much chance of conceiving.

Yet many IVF clinics are still not satisfied with these studies and so are not routinely recommending DHEA. To understand why there is such a divide and choose which side you agree with, it is useful to understand what the studies have found so far. But first, we need to identify who is likely to benefit from DHEA.

Who Should Consider Taking DHEA?

Most of the research on DHEA has focused on women with a condition called "diminished ovarian reserve." This condition is a major cause of failed IVF cycles, particularly in older women. Women with diminished ovarian reserve have exceptionally low success rates in IVF — by some measures, as low as 2–4%.[12]

Part of the problem is that as women reach their mid- to late 30s, the pool of follicles recruited each month to begin maturing shrinks in number. As a result, the number of eggs that can be stimulated by medication and then retrieved in an IVF cycle declines. This becomes a limiting factor to IVF success rates for women in their late 30s and 40s, and women over 40 are universally assumed to have diminished ovarian reserve.

For reasons that are not fully understood, diminished ovarian reserve also sometimes affects much younger women, in which case the term "premature ovarian aging" is sometimes used. In younger women, the condition is often diagnosed by measuring the level of a hormone called AMH, which reflects the number of follicles in very early stages of maturing. The results of an AMH test, together with the follicle count by ultrasound, predict how many eggs will likely be retrieved during an IVF cycle.

If your fertility specialist expects to retrieve only a small number of eggs, you may be diagnosed with diminished ovarian reserve.

Women with diminished ovarian reserve often overlap with the group of patients called "poor responders," in which the ovaries do not respond as expected to stimulation medication in an IVF cycle, and very few mature eggs are retrieved.

Poor responders and women with diminished ovarian reserve or premature ovarian aging typically have very low success rates in IVF, and cycles are often canceled because there are not enough eggs to retrieve. Research on DHEA has focused on these particular patients because this type of infertility is incredibly difficult to treat and DHEA appears to get at the core of the problem by increasing the number of eggs produced in an IVF cycle.

Based on current research, fertility specialists typically only recommend DHEA if you have been diagnosed with diminished ovarian reserve, you are over the age of 40 (some clinics say 35), or have had an IVF cycle that produced very few eggs. If you fall into one of these groups, DHEA may significantly improve your chance of conceiving, as described in the research that follows.

The Clinical Studies on DHEA

After witnessing extraordinary results in their first patient taking DHEA, the fertility specialists at CHR in New York began an initial study to find out whether DHEA could offer the same benefit to other women with diminished ovarian reserve who had little hope of producing enough eggs for a successful IVF cycle.

The group gave DHEA supplements to 25 patients with diminished ovarian reserve who were planning IVF. At the end of the IVF cycle, the resulting egg and embryo numbers were compared to each woman's previous IVF cycle without DHEA.[13] The results were impressive, showing increases in egg and embryo numbers along with improved egg quality.

This initial study was then followed up with a larger study in which women with diminished ovarian reserve were given DHEA for 4 months and the IVF outcomes compared to controls. In this study, the beneficial effects of DHEA on egg and embryos were again clearly apparent and translated into much higher pregnancy rates. Specifically, 28% of DHEA-treated women became pregnant, compared to just 10% of controls.[14]

Since that time, many other studies by the same group have confirmed that women with diminished ovarian reserve taking DHEA supplements before IVF have increased numbers of eggs and embryos, and higher pregnancy rates.

While the fertility specialists at CHR in New York pioneered the research into the ability of DHEA to improve outcomes in women with diminished ovarian reserve, other groups have reported similar positive results.[15] For example, a group in Turkey reported that DHEA treatment improved IVF pregnancy rates for poor responders from 10.5% to 47.4%.[16] The authors concluded that "DHEA supplementation might enhance ovarian response, reduce cycle cancellation rates and increase embryo quality in poor responders."

In 2010, a group in Israel reported the results from the first "randomized" clinical study using DHEA for poor responders undergoing IVF.[17] Half the women were randomly assigned to receive DHEA, while the other half did not. In the DHEA group, the women took the supplement for at least 6 weeks (if they conceived in the first cycle), or at least 16–18 weeks, through a second IVF cycle. At the end of the 2 cycles, the study revealed a significantly higher live-birth rate in the group taking DHEA: 23% versus 4%. The DHEA group also showed improved embryo quality over time. Although this was a small study, it provides further evidence that DHEA could be helpful for some women undergoing IVF.

In a second randomized clinical trial, published in 2013, both the doctors and patients were unaware of whether a particular patient was taking DHEA or a placebo (that is, the study was "double-blind"). This kind of study is designed to rule out any placebo effect or bias that could otherwise compromise the results. After three to four months, the group taking DHEA was found to have a significantly higher number of developing follicles, indicating that more eggs would be available for an IVF cycle.[18]

DHEA also appears to boost pregnancy chances even without IVF. Fertility specialists in Toronto reported positive results of treating women with DHEA for several months before IUI in conjunction with Clomid treatment. Compared to controls, DHEA-treated women showed higher follicle counts and improved pregnancy rates, with 29.8% conceiving versus 8.7% in the non-treated group, and a live birth rate of 21.3% versus 6.5%.[19] Researchers have also reported surprising numbers of naturally conceived pregnancies in women taking DHEA while waiting for IVF.

A group of doctors in Italy were so intrigued by the number of women conceiving spontaneously while taking DHEA that they decided to conduct a study to specifically investigate this phenomenon. In a paper published in 2013, the doctors reported that from a group of 39 younger "poor responders" taking DHEA for 3 months before starting IVF, 10 of these women became pregnant naturally before the IVF cycle began.[20]

The same phenomenon was also seen in women over 40, with 21% conceiving while taking DHEA in preparation for IVF, compared to just 4% of women in the control group. This is an extraordinary finding that requires further confirmation, but it is in line with anecdotal reports from several other fertility clinics.[21] If correct, these results indicate that DHEA may improve fertility enough for some women with diminished ovarian reserve to conceive even without IVF.[22]

DHEA and Miscarriage

DHEA does not just increase the number of eggs and embryos; it also appears to boost live birth rates by reducing chromosomal abnormalities in eggs and thereby preventing miscarriages. A study of IVF patients in two independent fertility clinics in New York and Toronto reported a substantial reduction in miscarriage rates in women taking DHEA.[23] In this study, pregnancy loss was reduced by 50–80% in comparison to national U.S. IVF pregnancy rates, bringing the miscarriage rate down to just 15% of pregnancies.

This low miscarriage rate is all the more surprising since women with diminished ovarian reserve are known to have much higher miscarriage rates than women with other causes of infertility.[24] After treatment with DHEA, the miscarriage rate dropped to the normal level seen in women without diminished ovarian reserve.[25]

Miscarriage rates are thought to be so high in women with diminished ovarian reserve because the vast majority of eggs are chromosomally abnormal ("aneuploid"). The CHR group noted that DHEA appears to decrease miscarriage rates to a degree that cannot be explained without a significant reduction of chromosomal abnormalities.[26] In other words, it would be mathematically impossible to reduce miscarriage rates to just 15% without reducing aneuploidy rates.

The CHR group then set out to delve into that question

a little further by looking at data from women who underwent IVF and had their embryos screened for chromosomal abnormalities. Within this patient population, the researchers identified a group of women with diminished ovarian reserve treated with DHEA and matched them to a control group that did not receive DHEA treatment.

Because diminished ovarian reserve is associated with very high levels of aneuploidy, one would expect much higher rates of aneuploidy in the diminished ovarian reserve group than in controls, but instead the reverse happened. In the control group, 61% of embryos were chromosomally abnormal, whereas only 38% of embryos from DHEA-treated women with diminished ovarian reserve were chromosomally abnormal.[27] This study provides preliminary evidence that DHEA supplements reduce the rate of chromosomal abnormalities, which explains why DHEA could have such a powerful impact on miscarriage rates.

This dramatic finding has been met with much skepticism, but if true, the reduction in chromosomal abnormalities after DHEA treatment actually has much wider implications for the way we understand egg quality and age-related infertility. It suggests that the increase in chromosomal abnormalities with age and diminished ovarian reserve are not a foregone conclusion; external factors such as hormones can, to some extent, correct the problem.

How Does DHEA Work?

DHEA is a molecule naturally produced in the body, and adequate levels are necessary for the production of certain hormones that are critical to fertility, including estrogen and testosterone. It appears that as we age, DHEA levels decline, thereby depriving the ovaries of vital hormones that help eggs develop properly.

By providing additional DHEA in the form of a supplement, it may be possible to make the ovaries function more like those of younger women, allowing more eggs to mature and improving egg quality.

Researchers have confirmed that DHEA supplements do in fact increase the levels of hormones and growth factors within the ovaries.[28] (This is why DHEA is not recommended for women with PCOS or a history of hormone-sensitive cancers). DHEA has specifically been found to promote the growth of very early-stage follicles — those follicles a couple of months away from ovulation.[29] It is thought to increase the number of eggs available for an IVF cycle by either increasing the pool of follicles that enter the early phase of maturing or increasing the proportion that survive these early stages without dying off.[30]

The fact that DHEA can reduce the rate of chromosomal abnormalities also suggests that chromosomal abnormalities are not a foregone conclusion in older women. Instead, aging may just create an environment in which an egg is predisposed to process chromosomes incorrectly in the months before ovulation.

DHEA could boost pregnancy rates in part by correcting the environment that the eggs mature in, increasing the chance that eggs will be able to process chromosomes correctly as they mature. This in turn could increase the number of eggs with normal chromosomes.[31]

One possible way that DHEA could encourage correct

processing of chromosomes is by boosting mitochondrial function, just as we saw in the discussion of Coenzyme Q10.[32] There is a solid scientific rationale for how increased mitochondrial function can increase the ability of eggs to process chromosomes correctly.[33] But whether DHEA does in fact assist mitochondria remains to be proven.

The Controversy

Given the very significant body of evidence showing the benefits of DHEA in improving egg and embryo numbers and quality, increasing pregnancy rates, and reducing miscarriage rates, you may be wondering why DHEA is still plagued by controversy.

The fact is that while a substantial proportion of IVF clinics are now routinely recommending DHEA for all women with diminished ovarian reserve, many clinics are not because they still regard DHEA as "experimental."[34] Even after a decade of positive research findings regarding DHEA, some experts have concluded that "its wide scale use cannot be currently recommended."[35]

The major criticism of the research on DHEA centers on the design of the studies. Specifically, critics claim that DHEA should not be recommended to patients yet because there have not been any large double-blind placebo-controlled trials. These are the "gold standard" clinical trials typically used for pharmaceutical drug approval.

Most studies to date have compared DHEA treatment to each woman's previous IVF cycle or to a matched group of patients not taking DHEA, rather than randomly assigning a large group of women to take DHEA or the placebo, with both doctor and patients unaware of which patients are taking which. Those few studies that have randomized patients to receive DHEA or a placebo have also been criticized as being too small and preliminary to change advice to patients.

Yet as the CHR group pointed out, it is extremely difficult to conduct a large, randomized placebo-controlled trial in this context because women with diminished ovarian reserve are often running out of time to get pregnant and are not willing to be randomly assigned to a placebo if there is a supplement available that could improve their chances. Several clinical trials had to be abandoned for this precise reason.[36]

The CHR group argues that the decision to use DHEA should be made based on the best available evidence rather than disregarding what we know so far while waiting for a study that meets the ideals of a gold-standard clinical trial.[37] Others disagree and maintain that DHEA cannot be recommended for routine use until its benefits have been proven in larger, more rigorous clinical studies.[38]

Refusing to recommend supplements in the absence of the type of clinical trial required for pharmaceutical drug approvals reflects a desire to ensure safety and effectiveness before patients waste time and money taking a supplement that does little to help. But when taken too far, this approach also denies patients treatments that have been shown to be safe and effective by numerous studies, albeit studies with some risk of bias and placebo effect.

History has shown that when concerns about bias or placebo effect are overestimated, patients can suffer. The controversy over folic acid serves as just one example: initial research showing that folic acid could prevent birth defects was blighted by the same type of criticism, leading to many years of heated controversy.[39]

Thirty years after the initial discovery of folic acid's benefits, we know that the early doubts about the value of folic acid in preventing birth defects probably caused many tragic outcomes that could have been avoided if medical advice had kept pace with research.

If DHEA is as beneficial as the current research indicates, questioning the value of this supplement may deprive some women of the opportunity to conceive with their own eggs or may incur the financial, emotional, and financial burden of repeating entire IVF cycles countless times to conceive when the odds of success are very low. And while most of the publications describing the benefits of DHEA come from only a small number of fertility clinics, the publications do consistently show a benefit for women with diminished ovarian reserve.

There is also a notable lack of research contradicting the positive findings of the studies described above. One of the only exceptions is a study suggesting that higher DHEA levels inside follicles are associated with lower egg and embryo quality.[40] But this finding is inconsistent with the other research showing significantly improved IVF outcomes, and almost every publication describing the use of DHEA before IVF has shown a clear benefit. The current research as a whole strongly suggests that DHEA represents a breakthrough for women with diminished ovarian reserve.

The IVF clinic that started the DHEA movement — CHR — has been routinely recommending DHEA for all patients with diminished ovarian reserve since 2007. [41] This means that women with low AMH or high FSH, or women over 40, typically take DHEA for at least two months, continuing through the stimulation phase of an IVF cycle. Many other IVF clinics also routinely recommend that DHEA should be offered to women with diminished ovarian reserve preparing for IVF.[42]

Safety and Side Effects

Because DHEA is thought to increase testosterone, it may have side effects related to male hormones, including oily skin, acne, hair loss, and facial hair growth.[43] Although some researchers have suggested that DHEA use may result in impaired insulin sensitivity, impaired glucose tolerance, liver problems, manic episodes, and other rare side effects,[44] these side effects have not been seen in the studies testing DHEA in the fertility context.

The CHR group has reported that in over a thousand patients supplemented with DHEA, they have not encountered a single complication of clinical significance.[45] The most commonly reported side effect among the patients at CHR taking DHEA was increased energy.[46] The randomized clinical study performed in Israel also found no significant side effects,[47] and additional studies outside the fertility context have reported that long-term use of DHEA is safe.[48]

Formulation and Dosing

If you decide to take DHEA, the specific formulation you buy could be important. While DHEA is readily available in pharmacies as a vitamin supplement, the purity and potency of formulations sold as supplements are quite inconsistent. Analysis of several brands has found that the actual DHEA dose can range from 0–150% of the labeled dose.[49]

Researchers have also discovered that it is important to use DHEA formulated in tiny microparticles to allow for absorption. This is called a "micronized" formulation.[50] Fertility clinics typically recommend that patients obtain pharmaceutical grade, micronized DHEA rather than buying one of the brands sold alongside vitamin supplements.

One option is the formulation used in several successful clinical trials, which is sold online as Fertinatal. According to the manufacturer, this formulation is potency guaranteed, micronized, pharmaceutical grade DHEA. Fertinatal is much more expensive than other DHEA supplements (at time of writing, a four-week supply costs $75) but may be a worthwhile investment if you choose to take DHEA because you are more likely to get the correct dose and a formulation that can actually be absorbed and have an effect, potentially saving the cost of a repeated IVF cycle. If Fertinatal is beyond your budget, look for another brand that says "micronized" on the label.

The dose of DHEA most often recommended by fertility clinics and used in clinical studies is 25 mg, three times per day.[51] Because studies have so consistently used this dose, there is very little research about what dose is actually needed to have a beneficial effect, and it may in fact be less. If you are undecided about whether you want to take DHEA or are concerned about cost, one option is to take a less frequent dose, such as 25 mg once or twice per day.

The research on DHEA suggests that it may take several months for this supplement to have a beneficial effect. For many women, this raises the question of whether or not to start taking DHEA if an IVF cycle is scheduled for just a few weeks away. This is a difficult decision and one to discuss with your doctor, but a factor to keep in mind is that if you do start taking DHEA and your upcoming cycle fails, you may at least have a better chance of the next IVF cycle succeeding because by that time, you will have been taking DHEA for the recommended two or three months.

Conclusion

If you have been diagnosed with diminished ovarian reserve or age-related infertility, consider taking a DHEA supplement for three months before your next IVF cycle to improve egg numbers and quality. Dr. Gleicher reports extraordinarily successful results from the use of DHEA in patients attending his clinic: "Over 90% of our DHEA patients have come to us from other programs with a recommendation for egg donation. They are not only women with diminished ovarian reserve, they are women with horribly diminished ovarian reserve — and still we have a third of them getting pregnant. It's remarkable."[52]

CHAPTER 10

Supplements That May Do More Harm Than Good

"If you trust Google more than your doctor then maybe it's time to switch doctors."

— JADELR AND CRISTINA CORDOVA

ONE OF THE natural consequences of the medical community's failure to give women complete information on which supplements may improve egg quality is that women must turn to less reliable sources of information and often end up taking supplements that are not supported by any scientific evidence.

This book features a vast number of clinical and laboratory studies showing that certain supplements can improve fertility, but attention must also be given to the supplements many women are taking in the hope of improving egg quality that are either ineffective or unsafe, or that may actually worsen egg quality and fertility.

Pycnogenol

Pycnogenol is a patented extract from pine bark that has been shown to have antioxidant properties. This antioxidant capacity has led some people to include pycnogenol on lists of supplements for egg quality, even though no evidence exists from any good-quality clinical trials. Because pycnogenol is a mixture of compounds not naturally found in the body, there is reason to be very cautious about its safety.

At the time of writing, there have not been any good-quality clinical studies showing that pycnogenol can improve egg quality or even that it is safe and lacks side effects. The company that makes pycnogenol, which has a website touting 40 years of research into this supplement, identifies countless studies on the use of pycnogenol for a variety of conditions, including male infertility, but not a single study on egg quality or female fertility.[1]

Given the lack of evidence, there is no reason to take pycnogenol when other much better antioxidant supplements are available to improve egg quality, such as CoQ10, vitamin E, and alpha-lipoic acid. These antioxidants are naturally found inside ovarian follicles, and their supplement forms have been widely studied for safety and side effects in many large, double-blind, placebo-controlled clinical trials.

Royal Jelly

Royal jelly is a substance secreted by worker bees to provide food for the queen bee. This jelly is thought to contain hormones that make the queen bee extremely fertile and increase her lifespan. Based on this natural role, royal jelly has long been recommended as an alternative medicine in the fertility context. Just like pycnogenol, royal jelly is a mixture of compounds not naturally found in the human body.

At the time of writing, no good-quality clinical research supports the use of royal jelly in improving egg quality, and it has been found to occasionally cause life-threatening allergic reactions. These allergic reactions likely occur because royal jelly contains some of the same allergens found in bee venom.[2] In addition, because royal jelly contains a mixture of chemicals that act like hormones, it may have unpredictable effects and disrupt natural hormone balance.[3] Given the uncertain benefit and side effects, royal jelly cannot be recommended as part of a regime to naturally improve fertility.

L-Arginine

L-arginine is another supplement that many women take in an effort to improve egg quality before IVF. Unlike pycnogenol and royal jelly, it is naturally found in the fluid of ovarian follicles, but that does not mean that taking extra in supplement form is necessarily beneficial for egg quality.

The theory behind using L-arginine to improve egg quality is that it increases the production of nitric oxide, which dilates blood vessels and therefore would be expected to increase blood flow to the ovaries and uterus, bringing with it hormones and nutrients that encourage follicles to grow.[4]

In one of the early studies aimed at improving IVF outcomes using L-arginine, the supplement did have the intended effect of improving blood flow.[5] In that study, L-arginine supplements were given to women who were considered "poor responders" in IVF. Poor responders are typically those who have a history of IVF cycles in which not enough follicles mature after IVF stimulation medication, leading to canceled and failed IVF cycles. This condition is thought to be caused by declining egg numbers and quality, often due to age.[6]

When 17 poor responders were given L-arginine during an IVF cycle and compared to poor responders not receiving arginine, it appeared that the supplement was beneficial. In the women taking L-arginine, fewer cycles were canceled, and an increased number of eggs were retrieved and embryos transferred. There were three pregnancies in the group taking L-arginine and no pregnancies in patients who did not take L-arginine; however, all three pregnancies resulted in early miscarriage — a clear sign that something may have been wrong with the quality of the eggs and embryos. Nevertheless, the authors concluded that L-arginine supplements may improve pregnancy rate in poor responders, who often have impaired blood flow.[7]

While this research seemed to bring good news, follow-up research by some of the same doctors a few years later revealed that L-arginine supplements may actually decrease egg and embryo quality. Unlike the first study, the follow-up study involved women with tubal infertility rather than poor responders. The researchers thought that L-arginine would offer the same benefits seen in poor responders by improving blood flow during IVF.

What they found was very unexpected. The women who received L-arginine instead of a placebo actually had fewer good-quality embryos and a lower chance of becoming pregnant.[8] The pregnancy rate per cycle was nearly halved (16.6% versus 31.6%), as was the pregnancy rate per embryo transfer (18.7% versus 37.5%). Embryo quality, measured based on the appearance of the embryo, was also negatively affected by L-arginine.

This research demonstrated that L-arginine supplements can significantly decrease egg and embryo quality. This decrease was thought to be caused by the very increase in permeability that was originally thought to make L-arginine beneficial. But instead of improving the conditions for follicle growth, this increase in permeability allowed hormones to get into the follicles too easily and too early in the egg development process, resulting in quick, intense, and inconsistent follicle growth.

One of the goals of IVF is to have a group of follicles mature steadily at the same time so that on the day of egg retrieval, they are all at the right stage of maturation and are ready to be fertilized. It may be that L-arginine causes some follicles to mature too quickly and chaotically.

Studies have also shown that nitric oxide, which is elevated after L-arginine supplementation, can decrease the level of cellular energy (ATP) and also increase the level of oxidizing molecules, both of which would be expected to damage eggs and embryos.[9] The doctors responsible for the study concluded that L-arginine supplements have a detrimental effect on embryo quality and the chance of becoming pregnant.

This result was probably not evident in their previous study with poor responders because the poor responders likely already had lower-than-normal nitric oxide levels, so L-arginine had the effect of bringing nitric oxide levels up to normal. Yet when this supplement was given to people with normal levels, L-arginine was very detrimental.

Even in the previous studies on poor responders showing an increase in egg numbers, the eggs may have all been very poor quality because each of the resulting pregnancies ended in early miscarriage.

More recent research by a separate group has confirmed the link between L-arginine and poor egg and embryo quality. In this research, instead of giving women L-arginine supplements, researchers measured the level of L-arginine naturally found in the fluid of ovarian follicles in 100 women undergoing IVF.[10]

The study revealed a strong link between higher L-arginine levels in ovarian follicles and fewer eggs retrieved and fewer embryos. The women in this study had a variety of causes of infertility, including male factor infertility, damaged or blocked fallopian tubes, endometriosis, and unexplained infertility. The clear implication from this research is that a high level of L-arginine has a negative effect on the development of eggs and embryos. Yet another study found that high nitric oxide levels are associated with implantation failure and fragmented embryos.[11]

With this research in mind, the only circumstance in which you should even consider taking L-arginine is if you have been diagnosed as a poor responder and have had multiple failed IVF cycles due to an insufficient number of eggs maturing. Even then, there is very limited evidence that L-arginine can improve egg numbers in poor responders, and this supplement may actually decrease egg quality. In anyone other than a poor responder, the evidence shows that L-arginine can reduce egg and embryo numbers and quality and is therefore not a recommended supplement.

Conclusion

Current scientific research provides no basis for taking pycnogenol, royal jelly, or L-arginine for the purpose of improving fertility. Many women are taking these supplements in the hope of improving egg quality or egg numbers, but to date there is little evidence of safety or efficacy. These unproven supplements may actually exacerbate the problem of poor egg quality, particularly in the case of L-arginine.

Part 3
THE **BIGGER** PICTURE

CHAPTER 11

The Egg Quality Diet

*"We are indeed much more than what we
eat, but what we eat can nevertheless help us
to be much more than what we are."*

— ADELLE DAVIS

To MANY, IT will come as no surprise that diet can have a powerful influence on fertility. Numerous books have been written on the subject, but unfortunately this abundance of nutritional advice is typically based on general ideas of a "healthy diet" rather than solid scientific research. When we delve into the actual research on how diet impacts fertility, some surprising patterns emerge.

This chapter begins with the most powerful change you can make to your diet — a switch to slowly digested carbohydrates instead of refined carbohydrates. This first step is critical to boosting egg quality and fertility.

Carbohydrates and Fertility

One of the key goals of a fertility diet is to balance your blood sugar and insulin levels by choosing the right kinds of carbohydrates. To understand why some carbohydrates are bad for fertility, we need to briefly delve into what happens when we eat carbohydrates.

After consuming refined carbohydrates such as white bread, the starches are quickly broken down by enzymes in the digestive system. Because starch is nothing more than long chains of glucose molecules joined end to end, when starch is digested, the glucose is released into the bloodstream, triggering a rapid rise in blood glucose levels.

In refined carbohydrates, in which the grain has been broken apart and pulverized into tiny particles to make flour, the starch molecules are easily accessible to digestive enzymes, so they can be broken down very quickly.

By contrast, unrefined grains and seeds such as quinoa take much longer to break down because the starches are still wrapped up inside the grain or seed. As a result, the starches are digested more slowly, and the glucose molecules are released gradually over time. This means that the blood sugar response after eating whole, unrefined grains is much slower and steadier. Instead of a sudden spike in glucose levels, there is a slow climb.

One of the problems with a sudden spike in blood glucose levels is that it causes the pancreas to release a huge amount of insulin in an effort to get muscle cells to take up glucose from the bloodstream. This system is important because if all the extra glucose stayed in the bloodstream, it would quickly cause damage throughout the body. Limb amputations in people with poorly controlled diabetes are the most dramatic example of this damage. The glucose needs to be safely stored away inside muscles or converted into fat. Insulin directs this process by telling muscle and fat cells to soak up glucose.

The higher the blood glucose level, the more insulin is released. Often, after a quick burst of glucose, the insulin response overshoots, causing blood glucose levels to drop too low. This then triggers cravings for another hit of quick-release carbohydrates, starting the whole cycle again.

Over time, with repeated high levels of sugar and insulin, the cells become resistant to insulin's message to soak up glucose, a condition called "insulin resistance." Blood glucose levels remain high, the body compensates by making even more insulin, and chaos ensues.

All this sugar and insulin is a big problem for fertility because it disrupts the balance of other hormones that regulate the reproductive system. It comes as a surprise to many people that insulin is a hormone that not only regulates glucose uptake and metabolism, but also regulates reproduction by binding to receptors in the ovaries and altering levels of other reproductive hormones.

For example, too much insulin leads to too much testosterone and other related "male" hormones. Many researchers now believe that this hormonal imbalance is the underlying cause of PCOS, one of the most common causes of infertility. As a result, PCOS serves as a clear example of how insulin can reduce fertility, and it is useful to understand this condition, even if you are not affected by PCOS.

One of the ways in which insulin function is disrupted in

many people with PCOS is that the muscles are "resistant" to insulin's message to take up glucose because there is a defect in the communication pathway. The practical result is that insulin does not function properly to tell the muscles to take up glucose, so more and more insulin is produced in an effort to get blood sugar under control.

While the muscles are not responding to insulin as they should, the insulin receptors in the ovaries use a different communication pathway that still works perfectly well. As a result, the ovaries respond easily to insulin's message to alter hormone production, only now there is vastly more insulin than normal, so hormone production in the ovaries is severely disrupted. This hormonal disruption then interferes with ovulation and fertility.

By understanding this mechanism, it is easy to see how insulin levels that are higher than normal as a result of indulging in too many refined carbohydrates and sugars could also disrupt hormone production in the ovaries.

Research has now confirmed that blood sugar and insulin do not just impact fertility in women with PCOS; frequent high blood sugar also has a negative impact on fertility in otherwise healthy women.

How Insulin Disrupts Ovulation

One of the first studies showing how blood sugar levels harm fertility in healthy women was published in 1999 by a group of researchers in Denmark.[1] In 165 couples trying to conceive, the researchers looked at a marker of average blood sugar levels over the preceding 3–4 months.

They did this by measuring levels of glycosylated hemoglobin, abbreviated as A1C. Hemoglobin is a protein in red blood cells; "glycosylated" means that sugar molecules have been attached to it. A1C reflects average blood glucose levels because when blood glucose is high, sugar molecules get attached to the hemoglobin protein. The more sugar-coated hemoglobin in the blood, the higher blood sugar has been over the previous several months. For this reason, A1C is typically used as a measure of diabetes.

What the Danish researchers found in this fertility study was striking: Women with high but still normal A1C levels were only *half* as likely to get pregnant over six months compared to women with lower A1C levels. This meant that women who, over the previous three to four months, had slightly elevated blood sugar levels had significantly reduced fertility.

The women with high but still normal A1C levels also had hormonal changes that were similar to a mild version of the hormonal and reproductive changes in PCOS.[2] These results provide strong evidence that even mild elevations in blood sugar levels can disrupt the hormonal system that controls fertility.

This brings us to one of the most valuable sources of information on how nutrition affects fertility: the Nurses Health Study. This extraordinary study revealed several factors impacting fertility, the most powerful of which came from the type of carbohydrates in the diet. Before we discuss the specific findings of the Nurses Health Study, it is worth noting just how immense this study was.

The Nurses Health Study began in 1975 and followed thousands of nurses over several decades. It was originally designed to determine the long-term effects of birth control but quickly evolved into a much larger survey on the impact of lifestyle factors on health and disease, becoming one of the most comprehensive health studies ever performed.

In 1989, a second round of the Nurses Health Study was initiated in order to answer more detailed questions and explore specific health issues such as fertility — issues that could not be fully analyzed in the earlier part of the study. In this second round, more than 100,000 women participated. Every 2 years, these women answered detailed questions about their diet, exercise, and many other lifestyle factors, along with recording whether they got pregnant or had a miscarriage.

From this group of 100,000 women, scientists at the Harvard School of Public Health then selected a subgroup of more than 18,000 women who were trying to get pregnant and had not previously reported problems with infertility.[3] The researchers analyzed 8 years of data from this subgroup to develop a picture of how nutrition could affect fertility. They did so by separating the women into 2 further subgroups: those who reported having ovulatory infertility (infertility caused by irregular ovulation or failure to ovulate) and those who did not. The researchers then compared the dietary patterns between both groups.

At the end of all this analysis, the Nurses Health Study revealed that while the total amount of carbohydrates in the diet was not connected to ovulatory infertility, the *type* of carbohydrates was very important. Women who ate more of the quickly digested carbohydrates that rapidly raise blood sugar were 78% more likely to have ovulatory infertility than women who ate slowly digested carbohydrates. Specifically, the particular carbohydrates linked to the highest risk of infertility were cold breakfast cereals, white rice, and potatoes; whereas brown rice and dark bread were linked to a lower risk of infertility.

For the purposes of the study, carbohydrates were categorized as "slow" or "fast" based on the glycemic index. This is a measure of the rise in blood glucose levels over a specific time period after eating a specific amount of carbohydrates. A high-glycemic carbohydrate, which is typically highly refined, is thus a "fast" carbohydrate that raises blood sugar levels too much and too quickly. A low-glycemic carbohydrate, typically minimally processed, is a "slow" carbohydrate.

To better compare the different foods, the researchers analyzing the Nurses Health Study actually went one step beyond the glycemic index and categorized foods using the "glycemic load." The glycemic load is a refinement of the glycemic index that takes into account the fact that you have to eat vastly different amounts of different foods to get the same amount of carbohydrates.

For example, basmati rice is lower on the glycemic index than watermelon, which might lead you to expect the rice to have less impact on your blood sugar levels. In reality, in an actual serving size, rice would have a much greater impact on blood sugar levels because it has a higher total carbohydrate content, whereas watermelon is mostly water. The glycemic load is a much more useful measure because it reflects the impact of a normal serving size on blood sugar levels.

The dramatic finding of the Nurses Health Study was that women who followed a diet of low-glycemic/"slow" carbohydrates had a much lower rate of ovulatory infertility. Thus, by modifying your diet to choose slow carbohydrates such as unrefined grains over fast carbohydrates such as potatoes, you may be able to balance blood sugar and insulin levels and thereby rebalance fertility hormones.

The magnitude of the impact of blood sugar levels on fertility outcomes in all of these studies is shocking, but the general trend is not. We would naturally expect that higher blood sugar and insulin contribute to infertility because we know that people who have particularly high blood sugar and insulin levels are at much greater risk for a variety of fertility problems. It has been known for many years that diabetes and insulin resistance contribute to ovulation disorders, poor egg quality, lower IVF success rates, and an increased risk of miscarriage.[4]

Insulin resistance and high insulin levels are also very common characteristics of women with PCOS who do not ovulate, and ovulation can often be restored or significantly improved with drugs that improve insulin function. [5] Insulin resistance is also much more common in infertile women who have an ovulation disorder, even without PCOS.[6]

High insulin levels are thought to impair ovulation by disrupting the delicate balance of hormones in the ovaries. Specifically, insulin increases levels of "male" hormones, such as testosterone, that are normally present in the ovaries in very small amounts.[7] These hormones, collectively called "androgens," encourage early follicle development but can interfere with later stages of egg development.[8]

High levels of androgens cause many small follicles to start developing, but the eggs inside cannot mature properly, and as a result ovulation may not occur. The excess of androgen hormones such as testosterone is likely to also cause many other hallmarks of PCOS: acne, facial hair growth, and weight gain.

Research also demonstrates that this hormonal impact of insulin on fertility is not only relevant to PCOS but also occurs in a milder form in women who consume high-glycemic carbohydrates and have a history of high blood sugar.[9] Even in normal, healthy women, elevated insulin may therefore contribute to ovulatory infertility.

The good news is that restoring insulin function improves ovulation and fertility,[10] and people with PCOS often have a dramatic improvement in symptoms after gaining control over insulin levels.

But disrupted ovulation is not the only manifestation of the ways in which high insulin and glucose levels impact fertility. There is also a very significant impact on egg quality.

Insulin and Egg Quality

Research has shown that high blood sugar and insulin levels significantly decrease egg quality. This in turn reduces the proportion of embryos that can successfully implant in the uterus, reduces IVF success rates, and increases the risk of early pregnancy loss.

The impact of insulin on egg quality is particularly apparent in the IVF context, as researchers in Japan demonstrated in 2011. To investigate whether there was any link between higher blood sugar levels and the results of IVF cycles, the researchers tested blood sugar levels in 150 women with various types of infertility being treated at an IVF clinic.[11]

Rather than just looking at a snapshot of blood sugar at one particular point in time, or sugar-coated hemoglobin as used in the Danish study mentioned earlier, the Japanese group measured the levels of "advanced glycosylation end products," which are molecules that accumulate in the blood as a result of high blood sugar levels over time.

The Japanese researchers found that women with higher levels of these molecules had fewer eggs retrieved, fewer eggs fertilized, and fewer good-quality embryos. The pregnancy rate was also very different: 23% in women with normal levels of these markers of long-term blood sugar levels compared to just 3.4% in women with high levels, which indicated a history of high blood sugar.[12]

Importantly, this study was not testing women known to have a risk factor for insulin resistance but rather a variety of infertility causes, including tubal factor and unexplained infertility. This means that the results are likely relevant for all women trying to conceive, suggesting a general need to control blood sugar levels for optimal egg quality.

Delving further into the question of how exactly high blood sugar and insulin reduce egg quality brings us right back to the subject of earlier chapters: mitochondria. As explained in earlier chapters, mitochondria are the tiny power plants inside all our cells that produce energy in the form of ATP. ATP is critically important to egg development, and as a result, any disruption in mitochondrial function compromises the ability of eggs to mature and to process chromosomes properly.

Decreased mitochondrial function in eggs from older women is thought to be a major reason why eggs from older women have more chromosomal abnormalities, resulting in lower fertilization and implantation rates and high miscarriage rates.

Recent animal studies have shown that high blood sugar and insulin levels impair mitochondrial function.[13] This decreases ATP levels, which causes the cellular machinery that processes chromosomes to malfunction. We would therefore expect an increase in the rate of chromosomal abnormalities. Researchers have confirmed that eggs from diabetic mice are indeed much more likely to have an incorrect number of chromosomes.[14]

The discovery that insulin resistance is associated with significant damage to mitochondria and disrupted egg development explains why women with high insulin levels who are undergoing IVF are at an increased risk of impaired embryo development, implantation failure, and poor IVF success rates.

But there is one more factor to consider when it comes to insulin and fertility, and that is the risk of miscarriage.

Insulin and Miscarriage Risk

Although often missed by doctors, there is a clear link between insulin resistance and the risk of miscarriage. More than a decade ago, scientists revealed that the rate of insulin resistance in women with recurrent pregnancy loss was nearly three times higher than normal.[15] Although the precise mechanism for this link is not well understood, research shows that high blood sugar or high insulin levels can significantly increase the risk of miscarriage.[16]

Putting it All Together

The clear message of all this research is that out-of-control blood sugar and insulin levels are bad news for fertility — for *all* women trying to conceive. This is particularly evident from the Danish study's finding that women with high but still normal sugar-coated hemoglobin levels were only *half* as likely to get pregnant over six months compared to women with lower levels.[17]

Even if you have no reason to believe that you have one of the common conditions linked to very high insulin levels (PCOS, diabetes, metabolic syndrome, or obesity), all the research demonstrating how blood sugar and insulin levels contribute to infertility in these conditions is relevant because studies show that even mild elevations in blood sugar levels over time can decrease egg quality and fertility in much the same way, just to a lesser extent.

But there is good news, too. Now that we understand the negative impact of high insulin levels, we have the opportunity to make a significant difference to fertility by getting our insulin under control. Studies confirm that doing so improves ovulation, egg quality, and fertility.[18]

How to Choose Carbohydrates for Optimum Fertility

What is the best way of achieving this overarching goal of managing blood sugar and insulin levels to help you conceive? One option is a very low-carbohydrate diet, but this is not recommended because research has shown that this type of diet can be hard to follow long-term and may deprive the body of certain key nutrients. An easier and healthier approach is to carefully select the right carbohydrates: carbohydrates that are digested slowly and that only moderately raise blood sugar, preventing sudden bursts of insulin.

A good starting point for choosing carbohydrates is the glycemic index, and we know that a low-glycemic diet can very effectively prevent high blood glucose and improve insulin function.[19] While this provides a valuable starting point for choosing carbohydrates, the glycemic index does have some limitations because it underestimates the effect of simple sugars. As a result, to get the most benefit for fertility, we need to modify the traditional low-glycemic diet by carefully limiting all sugars, regardless of what the glycemic index tells us. But before we turn specifically to sugars, we start with the part of the diet where the glycemic index is most helpful: grains and starches.

To control your insulin levels, your general philosophy for grains should be to choose minimally processed whole grains such as quinoa, wild rice, beans, seeds, brown rice, and buckwheat over anything made from flour, such as bread, or processed into breakfast cereal.

The term "whole-grain" in food packaging can often be misleading. Real whole grains, which are broken down much more slowly and also carry more nutrients than refined grains, will still look like the original grain. This is very different from processed foods made with "whole-grain" flour, in which the nutrient-containing layers are stripped away, the rest of the grain has been pulverized into flour, and some of the nutrient-packed part of the grain is then added back in to make breakfast cereal or bread flour. This second type of "whole-grain" food is vastly inferior to actual whole grains because the grain is already broken down, so the carbohydrates are released more quickly and there is a greater impact on blood sugar.

To boost your fertility, you should minimize any highly processed grains such as bread and pasta, and choose high-fiber versions, such as bran cereal and wholemeal spaghetti, when you can.

Adopting this general approach of choosing unrefined whole grains and choosing high-fiber options when you do eat foods made from refined grains means you will not have to learn the glycemic load of individual foods. You will intuitively know that anything white and highly processed will raise blood sugar levels and should be avoided. But for illustration purposes, some examples of high- and low-glycemic carbohydrates are listed below:

High Glycemic Load: [20]

- corn flakes
- white bread
- bagel
- instant oatmeal
- white rice
- conventional pasta

Low Glycemic Load:

- pumpernickel bread
- quinoa
- couscous
- bran cereal (Kellogg's All-Bran, Raisin Bran)

- wholemeal spaghetti

- kidney beans

- lentils

- chickpeas

Yet glycemic load and the glycemic index do have a major shortcoming. They are only really useful for starchy or grain-based foods and fall short when it comes to sugar.

The Confusing World of Sugar

Although most people intuitively understand that eating sugar raises blood sugar, there is a lot of confusion about which sugars are particularly bad for you, as evident from the controversy over high-fructose corn syrup. The simple answer is that all sugar is problematic for fertility and egg quality.

Fructose and glucose are simple sugars, and both are found naturally in fruit in similar amounts. Table sugar, also called sucrose, is one molecule of fructose joined to one molecule of glucose. High-fructose corn syrup is similarly a mix of approximately equal amounts of fructose and glucose. The differences between the sugars found in fruit, honey, table sugar, and high-fructose corn syrup are minimal — all these sugars cause similar rises in blood sugar and insulin,[21] and so pose the same problem for fertility. And sugar is much worse than the glycemic index would lead you to believe. This is because the glycemic index virtually ignores the effect of fructose.

The glycemic index and glycemic load reflect the impact on just one sugar in the blood: glucose. As many nutritionists have observed in recent years, fructose has relatively little effect on blood glucose levels. So according to the glycemic index, agave syrup, which is 90% fructose, has very little impact on blood sugar and would theoretically be a healthy choice. Yet we must go one step further when it comes to fertility and think about insulin.

Insulin is a major reason we care about controlling blood glucose levels in a fertility diet because high levels of insulin interfere with fertility hormones. What the glycemic index ignores is the fact that fructose itself may not raise glucose much, but over time it contributes to high insulin levels.

Although fructose does not trigger the same immediate release of insulin from the pancreas, research has demonstrated that long-term consumption of large amounts of fructose interferes with insulin function and significantly raises insulin levels.[22] (As just one example, a study demonstrated that adding extra fructose to a person's diet for 10 weeks significantly increased fasting insulin levels, suggesting that fructose contributes to insulin resistance.)[23] As a result, large amounts of fructose have the clear potential to negatively affect fertility.

To maximize your fertility, it is important to be mindful of all sugars, whether in the form of regular sugar, high-fructose corn syrup, honey, or fruit. All these sources of sugar have roughly similar ratios of glucose and fructose, both of which are bad for fertility.

This does not mean that fruit and candy are on the same footing. Rather than focusing on the specific type of sugar, you should make food choices based on the nutritional payoff that comes along with sugar. For example, soda and other sugary drinks have no redeeming nutritional qualities — they raise blood sugar and insulin levels without making you feel full and without providing any vitamins or other nutrients. Fruit is quite different because all the vitamins, antioxidants, and fiber found naturally in fruit are beneficial for fertility and compensate for the impact on blood sugar.

Something to keep in mind when choosing fruit is that the glycemic index is not a reliable guide as to which fruits have less impact on your insulin levels. Lower-glycemic fruits are often just those that have a greater proportion of sugar in the form of fructose, which is ignored by the glycemic index.

The best plan is to limit your overall consumption of fruit to a few servings per day and choose fruits with a lower total amount of sugar and either a high-fiber content or a high anti-oxidant content, such as apples, pears, and berries.

If you have PCOS and therefore need to control your blood sugar levels even more closely, it may be wise to limit fruit to just one or two servings per day and make this the only significant source of sugar in your diet.

Do Vegetables Impact Blood Sugar?

Almost all vegetables are super-foods for fertility. The only ones to even pause over are starchy or sweet ones: potatoes, winter squash, pumpkin, sweet potatoes, carrots, yams, and corn. These vegetables will have a greater impact on blood sugar levels than other vegetables, but this impact is generally compensated for by the nutritional value they provide.

The exceptions here may be potatoes and corn, which each have a very significant impact on glucose levels and are much lower in antioxidants and nutrients than other vegetables. As a result, the nutritional value they provide is not worth the cost to blood sugar levels. By contrast, sweet potatoes, carrots, and pumpkin are rich in beta-carotene, a vitamin A precursor that is very important to fertility. These brightly colored vegetables are also rich in many other vitamins and so are good nutritional choices.

Other Benefits to Balancing Blood Sugar

A side benefit to cutting back on sugar and choosing slow carbohydrates over quick-release carbohydrates is that as a result of the steady levels of sugar and insulin rather than peaks and crashes, you will feel full longer and crave carbohydrates less. This is because the sudden bursts of insulin released to cope with high blood sugar levels will often drive blood glucose too low, leaving you craving another quick hit of carbohydrates.

In contrast, with a steady rise in blood glucose levels, the relatively small insulin response will not drive blood glucose levels down so far, minimizing the peaks and valleys in your blood sugar levels. Your mood, energy level, and food cravings will likely improve, and if you are overweight, this strategy will probably also help you lose weight without feeling hungry. This can itself be a huge benefit for fertility — just a 5–10% weight loss in overweight women can restore fertility.

Gluten-Free Carbohydrates

Before leaving the topic of carbohydrates, a word about the wave of new gluten-free bread, pasta, cake, and cookies available in supermarkets. Unless you have celiac disease or a wheat or gluten allergy, these gluten-free refined carbohydrates are not necessarily any healthier than traditional choices, and in many cases actually cause a more dramatic blood sugar spike.

Gluten is a protein found in wheat and a few other grains. In some people it triggers an autoimmune condition called celiac disease, which is very bad news for fertility. As discussed in chapter 4, if you have any symptoms of celiac disease and are struggling with infertility, it is a good idea to ask your doctor for a blood test to rule out this disease.

If you have celiac disease, eliminating gluten from your life could increase your chance of getting pregnant and significantly reduce your risk of miscarriage. But if you do not have celiac disease or a gluten intolerance, gluten-free foods are not necessarily healthier carbohydrates.

The Bottom Line on Carbohydrates

In short, to boost fertility, the best carbohydrates are minimally processed grains and vitamin-packed vegetables. When you do eat refined carbohydrates, choose high-fiber versions and minimize all forms of sugar. This plan will stabilize your blood sugar and insulin levels and thereby rebalance other hormones involved in fertility, giving you the best chance of becoming pregnant.

Trans Fat

Insulin resistance is not just a result of quick-release carbohydrates; another contributing factor could be a higher intake of trans fats. For this reason, avoiding trans fat is another important goal of a fertility diet.

Trans fats are most often found in commercial baked and

fried foods, such as doughnuts and cookies. They are man-made fats created to increase a product's shelf life and allow oil to be reused after it has been heated. As research emerged linking trans fats to a variety of health problems, government regulators in many jurisdictions stepped in and mandated labeling or strict limits on the allowed amount of trans fats. This led to a significant decrease in the use of trans fats, with major companies reformulating their products to reduce or eliminate trans fats. Some European countries have banned trans fats entirely, and the U.S. FDA has announced plans to follow suit. Yet in some countries, trans fats remain entirely unrestricted (at time of writing, the United Kingdom, for example).

Unfortunately, it doesn't take much trans fat to have a harmful effect. Even a few grams per day has been linked to an increased risk of type II diabetes, insulin resistance, cardiovascular disease, and inflammation. As a result of the Nurses Health Study, we know that trans fats also significantly increase the risk of infertility.

When analyzing trans fat intake in the Nurses Health Study data, the researchers at the Harvard School of Public Health found that consuming even a small amount of trans fat rather than monounsaturated fat was associated with a more than doubled risk of ovulatory infertility.[24]

Trans fats are thought to be so problematic for fertility because they decrease the activity of specific receptors involved in metabolism.[25] These receptors, called peroxisome proliferator activated receptor gamma (PPAR-gamma), are involved in insulin function. Several drugs designed to improve insulin function in diabetics and PCOS patients directly target these receptors to improve insulin function.[26] It appears that trans fats do the exact opposite, interfering with the function of these receptors. It is not surprising, then, that trans fats can contribute to poor insulin function, which we now understand can contribute to infertility.

The simple solution is to limit trans fats in your diet as much as possible. Trans fats have no redeeming nutritional qualities and are not typically found in healthy and natural food. There is no need to jeopardize your fertility with these artificial fats once you know how to avoid them.

If you live in a country where trans fats are permitted, you will need to carefully read product labels of any processed food you buy. A claim of "zero grams" of trans fat per serving on the label can be meaningless, so you have to go beyond the nutritional information and look at the product ingredients.

If you find "hydrogenated" or "partially hydrogenated" oil, this is code for trans fat. The reality is that most products containing trans fats also contain unhealthy refined carbohydrates that you should already be avoiding as part of a fertility diet, such as cookies, potato chips, doughnuts, and fast food. Cutting these processed, refined carbohydrates from your diet is an effective way to reduce your trans fat intake.

Boosting Fertility with a Mediterranean Diet

Beyond carbohydrates and trans fat, there is also a growing body of evidence showing how general dietary patterns can impact fertility. Diet surveys of women undergoing IVF or trying to conceive naturally have revealed that a diet based on vegetables, fruit, vegetable oils, legumes, and lean proteins (fish in particular), together with low-glycemic carbohydrates, dramatically improves fertility.

The Nurses Health Study is by far the largest and most detailed study to address the question of how overall diet impacts fertility. By studying the diets of thousands of women participating in the study while trying to conceive, researchers uncovered a group of specific dietary factors associated with a lower risk of infertility.

Specifically, the researchers found that the diet having the lowest risk of infertility was based on higher consumption of monounsaturated fatty acids, vegetable rather than animal protein sources, low-glycemic carbohydrates, and, somewhat unexpectedly, greater consumption of full-fat dairy. The women who closely followed this diet had a 60% lower risk of ovulatory infertility and a 27% lower risk of infertility due to other causes.

The Nurses Health Study therefore suggests that diet can go a long way toward preventing infertility caused by ovulatory disorders. But the focus on "ovulatory infertility" in this study is important to note. This type of infertility refers to women who have difficulty conceiving because they are not ovulating regularly, and PCOS is by far the most common cause of this disorder. From the Nurses Health Study alone, we cannot know whether other types of infertility, such as that caused by age or poor egg quality, may benefit from different dietary guidelines.

For greater understanding of how diet impacts these other causes of infertility, we have to go beyond the Nurses Health Study and look at research showing how diet impacts IVF success rates. This allows us to identify the diet that is most useful to women trying to conceive through IVF, in which egg quality is often the limiting factor.

One of the most interesting studies on diet and IVF success rates surveyed 161 couples at an IVF clinic in the Netherlands. After analyzing each woman's diet, researchers found that those women who closely followed a Mediterranean diet before their IVF cycle had a 40% higher chance of becoming pregnant.[27] The "Mediterranean diet" in this study was characterized by a high intake of vegetables, vegetable oil, fish, and legumes, and a lower intake of processed snacks.

The researchers weren't sure why this Mediterranean diet improved pregnancy rates so dramatically but suggested that it was a result of specific vitamins and fatty acids. This theory is strongly supported by the fact that women who closely followed the Mediterranean diet had significantly higher levels of folate (found in grains and vegetables), and also somewhat higher levels of vitamin B6 and vitamin B12 (found in fish, dairy, eggs, and meat).

Each of these vitamins benefits fertility in a number of ways, but their biggest impact could be through reducing levels of a harmful amino acid called homocysteine. The Dutch researchers found that the more closely women followed the Mediterranean diet, the lower their homocysteine levels.

As described in earlier chapters, scientists have known for many years that a deficiency in folate or vitamin B12 causes the amino acid homocysteine to build up in the body, which in turn reduces the number and quality of eggs in IVF cycles and reduces embryo quality.[28] High homocysteine levels have also been linked to a high rate of miscarriage.[29]

The Mediterranean diet may therefore improve pregnancy chances in IVF by increasing levels of key fertility vitamins and decreasing homocysteine, thereby improving egg and embryo quality.

Vitamin B6 alone could also have a major impact on boosting fertility in women following a Mediterranean diet because research has established that giving vitamin B6 supplements to women with infertility increases the chance of conception by 40% and decreases early miscarriage by 30%.[30] Vitamin B6 is found in particularly large amounts in fish, a key component of the Mediterranean diet.

If vitamins B6 and B12 are part of the reason for improved IVF success rates for women following a Mediterranean diet, the advice from the Nurses Health Study to choose vegetable protein over animal protein could be counterproductive. If egg quality is the limiting factor in your ability to get pregnant (if you are over 35 or have had failed IVF cycles, for example), getting adequate levels of vitamin B12 is important, and vitamin B12 is typically only found in animal foods. A deficiency of this vitamin is very common in vegetarians and particularly in vegans. [31] Vitamin B6 is also much easier to obtain from animal sources, such as fish, pork, and chicken.

In another useful study investigating the link between diet and pregnancy rates during IVF, women who met the Dutch nutritional guidelines for daily consumption of fruit, vegetables, meat, fish, and whole wheat products had much higher pregnancy rates.[32] The Dutch nutritional guidelines advise at least two pieces of fruit per day, at least 200 grams of vegetables, the use of monounsaturated or polyunsaturated oils, at least three servings of meat or meat replacers weekly, at least four slices of whole wheat bread per day, and at least one serving of fish per week. This diet generally corresponds to the Mediterranean diet, although perhaps with a greater focus on bread.

The researchers found that women who more closely followed the Dutch nutritional guidelines before their IVF cycle had a 65% higher chance of pregnancy. Again, researchers suspected that the effects of B vitamins such as folic acid could help explain how improved nutrition increases pregnancy rates.

Another possibility raised by researchers is that a Mediterranean diet is beneficial because it includes more of the healthy fats found in fish, nuts, and vegetable oils.[33] Evidence is emerging that some of the specific types of polyunsaturated fats that are emphasized in a Mediterranean diet have a positive impact on egg quality and fertility.

"Polyunsaturated" fats are those that have more than one double bond in their long molecular backbone, which gives each fat molecule a bent, crooked shape, so they cannot pack together closely and are therefore liquid at room temperature. Two groups of polyunsaturated fats are the omega-3 and omega-6 fatty acids. The "3" and "6" in this context refer to the position of the first double bond in these fats, and each is actually a group of different fats, with omega-3 fats including DHA and EPA, for example.

The typical modern diet has a much greater proportion of omega-6s than omega-3s, which is thought to contribute to inflammation throughout the body and is a risk factor underlying a variety of health conditions.

A separate study in the Netherlands addressed the specific question of the impact of polyunsaturated fatty acids and diet on IVF success rates. The study found that women with the highest levels of omega-3 fatty acids had improved embryo quality.[34] This fits with the traditional idea that omega-3 fatty acids are good and omega-6 fatty acids are bad, but the situation is in fact much more nuanced. Some omega-6 fatty acids are much worse than others.

The normal human diet is very high in a particular type of omega-6 fatty acid called linoleic acid. This is found in a wide variety of foods and is not regarded as posing much of a risk to health or fertility. By contrast, one of the most problematic omega-6 fatty acids, called arachidonic acid, has been linked to arthritis, asthma, allergies, heart disease, and diabetes.[35] The body makes small amounts of arachidonic acid from other types of omega-6 fatty acids, but most arachidonic acid in the body comes directly from food.

Some of the foods that contribute the most arachidonic acid to our diet are protein sources that are often considered healthy — including turkey and farmed salmon. Beef, lamb, and lean pork have relatively less arachidonic acid.

To further explore the question of which specific fatty acids impact fertility, researchers in Iran measured the levels of individual fatty acids in the follicle fluid of women undergoing IVF. The researchers found a few general trends that further supported the concept of the Mediterranean diet improving fertility.[36] Specifically, they found that women who became pregnant after IVF had a higher overall level of omega-3 fatty acids in their ovaries and a high proportion of omega-3 to omega-6.

As we would expect, not all omega-6 fatty acids were bad news for fertility in the Iranian study. But the "bad" omega-6 fatty acid, arachidonic acid, was linked to decreased fertility. Specifically, in women with higher arachidonic acid levels, their eggs were less likely to fertilize. Also, women who became pregnant had slightly lower arachidonic acid levels than women who did not.

Fatty acids could also explain one puzzling trend revealed in the Nurses Health Study, which suggested that replacing some animal sources of protein with vegetable sources may reduce the risk of ovulatory infertility. Replacing animal protein with vegetable protein may in fact reduce the levels of arachidonic acid because some animal proteins, such as turkey, have quite high levels of this fatty acid.

Further details of the Nurses Health Study provide some support for this explanation because the researchers found that fish had no impact on fertility, while increased consumption of turkey and chicken did slightly increase the risk of infertility. This is consistent with the idea that it may be the fatty acids in these protein sources that contribute to the infertility risk.

With the explanation of the differing effect of some animal proteins, we do not have to take the finding of the Nurses Health Study at face value and replace all animal protein with plant protein. Instead, we can choose the animal protein sources with a healthy balance of fatty acids, specifically those protein sources with the lowest amount of arachidonic acid and highest omega-3 levels. This means replacing turkey and dark-meat chicken with fish, chicken breast, grass-fed beef, lamb, and lean pork.

The exception to the rule here is farmed salmon. Although wild salmon and all other types of fish are low in harmful omega-6 fatty acids and high in omega-3s, farmed salmon is different. Because farmed salmon is typically fed corn and soy products instead of its natural diet, it is incredibly high in arachidonic acid. As a result, virtually every other low-mercury fish is a better choice for a fertility diet.

It goes without saying that you should avoid any high-mercury fish while trying to conceive. The fish highest in mercury are shark, swordfish, tilefish, and king mackerel.[37] Albacore tuna also contains a moderate amount of mercury and should not be eaten more than once per week. Canned light tuna is relatively low in mercury.

Piecing together the features of the general dietary patterns shown to benefit fertility in these studies, there are some clear common features:

- low-glycemic carbohydrates

- vegetables

- the polyunsaturated and monounsaturated fats found in the Mediterranean diet

The protein side of the equation is more complex, but with an understanding of the role of fatty acids and the need to get sufficient vitamins B6 and B12, we can refine the protein advice from the Nurses Health Study diet to more closely correspond to the Mediterranean diet and choose fish and other healthy animal protein sources.

This overall diet also happens to correspond to the anti-inflammatory diet shown to reduce the severity of arthritis, diabetes, heart disease, autoimmune diseases, and a variety of other specific diseases. Because the diet is so beneficial to overall health, much has already been written about the day-to-day details, and many recipe books are available.

For further reading, see:

- *The Inflammation Free Diet Plan*, by Monica Reinagel and Julius Torelli, M.D.
- *Win the War Within*, by Floyd Chilton, Ph.D.
- *The Blood Sugar Solution Cookbook*, by Mark Hyman, M.D.

Alcohol and Caffeine

There is some evidence that limiting your caffeine and alcohol consumption could be helpful to fertility, although research remains quite inconsistent.

Does Alcohol Harm Fertility?

It is clear that a high level of alcohol consumption has a noticeable impact on fertility,[38] but the evidence is much more ambiguous as to the impact of occasional alcohol consumption on the ability to conceive.[39] One factor that may have complicated research over the years is age, with a Danish study finding that alcohol intake was a significant predictor of infertility only among women over 30. In the over-30 age group, women consuming 7 or more alcoholic drinks per week were more than twice as likely to report infertility as women consuming less than 1 drink per week.[40]

A high-profile Danish study published in 1998 indicated that alcohol intake is associated with reduced fertility and increased time to pregnancy even among women drinking five or fewer alcoholic drinks per week.[41] Alcohol consumption has also been linked to ovulatory infertility in some studies but not others.[42]

Researchers have now also seen a negative effect of moderate alcohol consumption on IVF success rates. The first such study, published by researchers at the University of California in 2003, found that alcohol consumption in the month prior to IVF had a very significant effect on the chance of pregnancy, while alcohol consumption in the week before IVF doubled the miscarriage rate. Alcohol consumption was also associated with a decrease in the number of eggs retrieved.[43]

More recently, a larger study investigating the question of alcohol and IVF success rates confirmed a negative effect of alcohol, but the difference in success rates was much smaller than the previous research indicated. That study, published in 2011 by researchers at Harvard Medical School, was based on a survey of more than 2,000 couples undergoing IVF. The researchers found that compared to women reporting fewer than 4 alcoholic drinks per week, women drinking more than this amount had a 16% lower chance of a live birth.[44]

Even though the evidence is not entirely consistent on the impact of one or two alcoholic drinks per week, research does show that greater alcohol consumption is associated with a longer time to conceive and reduced IVF success rates. Since you will have to give up alcohol completely once pregnant anyway, it is probably worth starting earlier and reducing or eliminating alcohol while trying to conceive.

Caffeine and Fertility

The evidence is even less clear when it comes to caffeine. While high levels of caffeine consumption have been linked to much longer time to pregnancy and increased risk of miscarriage, many of these studies involved women drinking more than five or six cups of tea or coffee per day.[45] There is very little research showing a clear impact of just one or two cups per day while trying to conceive.

Nevertheless, a Yale study revealed that women who used to drink tea or coffee in the past, but stopped prior to fertility treatment, had a higher pregnancy and live birth rate than current tea and coffee drinkers.[46] Furthermore, one recent study measured caffeine levels inside ovarian follicles and demonstrated that caffeine does indeed reach the fluid inside the follicles. This study found no association between caffeine levels and pregnancy rate after IVF but did suggest a possible link between higher caffeine levels and early pregnancy loss, along with a decrease in the number of good-quality embryos.[47]

So while it is probably not necessary to stop drinking tea and coffee altogether, there is reason to be cautious about how much caffeine you are consuming. In the IVF context, there can be so much at stake in terms of financial cost, inconvenience, anxiety, and discomfort that you may be willing to give up caffeine just in case it makes a difference. But if that is not your philosophy, one cup of tea or coffee is probably not worth feeling guilty about.

The Overall Fertility Diet

Clear scientific evidence has established that certain types of carbohydrates harm fertility by causing spikes in blood sugar levels, which in turn cause major hormonal disruptions and reduce egg quality. Keeping blood sugar levels steady by choosing low-glycemic carbohydrates over refined starches and sugars can benefit anyone trying to have a baby, but it is particularly important if you have PCOS or diabetes.

Recent research has also revealed some general dietary patterns that are associated with improved fertility. Specifically, several researchers have discovered that women following a Mediterranean diet have higher success rates in IVF. There is very good reason for this: The Mediterranean diet emphasizes vegetables, healthy fats, lean meat, and seafood, all of which are higher in specific vitamins and fatty acids associated with improved fertility, and lower in the fatty acids and refined carbohydrates that cause inflammation and hormonal disruptions throughout the body, compromising fertility.

To boost your fertility, the best approach is to focus on choosing the right kind of carbohydrates, minimizing processed food, and following general dietary principles that maximize vitamins, antioxidants, and healthy fats.

Action Steps

To boost your fertility, choose a diet based on:

- Non-starchy, vitamin-packed vegetables such as spinach, bell peppers, kale, broccoli, and salad greens

- Lean, unprocessed protein such as fish, chicken, lean meat (preferably grass-fed), beans, and legumes

- Healthy fats such as olive oil, avocado, and nuts

- Limited amounts of whole, unrefined carbohydrates such as quinoa, wild rice, and buckwheat, and only refined carbohydrates that are high in fiber, such as bran cereal

- Berries and limited amounts of other fruit

- Limited amounts of starchy, brightly colored vegetables such as sweet potato, winter squash, pumpkin, and carrots

You can further improve your egg quality and fertility by avoiding or carefully limiting:

- "white" carbohydrates such as sugar, white bread, most breakfast cereals, pasta, and potatoes

- Processed foods containing trans fats

- Caffeine and alcohol

CHAPTER 12

The Other Half of the Equation: Sperm Quality

"The difference between the impossible and the possible lies in a man's determination."
— TOMMY LASORDA

MOST COUPLES WHO are trying to conceive are never told the basic facts about sperm quality and male fertility. This lack of information deprives men of the chance to take simple steps to improve their fertility — steps that are backed up by years of scientific research.

If a couple has difficulty conceiving due to poor sperm quality, the focus usually shifts to fertility treatments that can circumvent the issue rather than address it. A more rational approach is to tackle the underlying cause and find solutions for poor sperm quality. But first, we need to dispel some of pervasive myths surrounding male fertility.

Myth No. 1:
Difficulty conceiving can usually be attributed to the female partner

Contrary to popular belief, male infertility contributes to nearly 50% of all cases in which a couple has difficulty conceiving.[1] The misconception that female infertility is more common may be due to the fact that treatment in a fertility clinic typically entails many procedures, medications, and injections for women but not for men.

Even though the female partner is nearly always the main focus of fertility treatments such as IUI and IVF, in many cases these treatments are needed only to circumvent problems with sperm quality rather than any female fertility issues. Yet even with these advanced fertility treatments as a work-around, low sperm quality can remain a limiting factor and can increase the risk of miscarriage. In the end, whether a couple is trying to conceive naturally or through IVF, the male side of the equation should not be ignored.

Part of the problem is that traditional semen analysis done in fertility clinics is woefully inadequate. Three standard measures are analyzed during a conventional semen analysis (together termed "semen parameters"):

1. Sperm Count/Concentration: the number of sperm per unit of volume of semen

2. Motility: the sperm's ability to swim properly toward the egg

3. Morphology: the percent of sperm that have a
normal shape and overall appearance

While a problem in any one of these parameters will definitely make it more difficult to conceive, this traditional semen analysis does not tell the whole story. The screening may come back perfectly normal, even though poor sperm quality remains a barrier to conceiving. This is because the traditional measures do not adequately investigate the quality of the DNA inside the sperm.

The latest research suggests that DNA quality matters more than conventional semen parameters. The term "DNA quality" reflects whether the DNA has individual mutations, extra or missing copies of chromosomes, or physical breaks in the DNA strands. This last type of damage results in fragmentation of the chromosomes and is the type of damage most often used to measure DNA quality in sperm.

Each type of damage to DNA causes its own set of problems: decreased chance of fertilization, decreased chance of the embryo successfully implanting to become a pregnancy, and increased risk of the child being born with a serious birth defect or a genetic disease caused by a new spontaneous mutation.

Evidence is emerging that DNA damage in sperm also increases the risk of miscarriage. In one recent study, researchers found much higher levels of DNA damage in sperm from couples with a history of unexplained miscarriage, suggesting that this DNA damage could be a contributing factor to pregnancy loss.[2]

In short, the extent of DNA damage in sperm is an important factor for any couple trying to conceive.

Myth No. 2:
Male fertility does not decline until after age 50

The reality is that a typical 45-year-old man is significantly less fertile than a man 10 years younger, with sperm quality beginning to decline as early as age 35.[3] A large part of the reason for this decline is that sperm from older men have more DNA breakage, DNA mutations, and other chromosomal abnormalities.[4] In fact, DNA fragmentation in sperm doubles from ages 30–45.[5]

The age-related decline in male fertility is often overlooked. Many people wrongly assume that while an older mother is more likely to miscarry or have a baby with a birth defect such as Down's syndrome, the father's age has no impact on these outcomes. Research shows that fathers over the age of 40 have a 20% greater chance of having a baby with a serious birth defect.[6] And as a result of the DNA errors that increase with age, men over 50 are twice as likely to have a child with autism when compared with men under 29.[7] Higher levels of DNA damage in sperm also more than double the risk of miscarriage. [8]

It is not just the DNA inside sperm that suffers with increasing age. Sperm motility starts to decline at age 35, and age also negatively impacts sperm count and morphology.[9]

But it's not all bad news. Research also shows that some of this decline can be prevented and reversed, with several studies finding that older men following a healthy diet and taking the right supplements have sperm quality similar to younger men. This brings us to the most significant myth of all.

Myth No. 3:
Nothing can be done to improve sperm quality

Decades of scientific research contradict this widely held belief and show that it is possible to improve sperm quality and even improve the quality of the DNA within the sperm. Doing so has a whole host of benefits: increasing the chance of conceiving (whether naturally or in conjunction with assisted reproduction such as IVF) and reducing the risk of miscarriage and birth defects.

To understand what you can do to improve sperm quality, it helps to first understand how sperm become damaged in the first place.

The cycle of producing each sperm takes a little over two months.[10] During this time, many different environmental and lifestyle factors can impact the process, for better or worse. Yet by far the most important factor impacting sperm quality during this time is the level of oxidation.

Oxidation is a chemical reaction in the body that is analogous to metal rusting or an apple turning brown. As sperm are produced, a normal, healthy level of oxidation takes place as a result of biological processes, and an army of defenders stop this oxidation from getting out of control. The defense system includes antioxidants such as vitamins C and E (semen contains a particularly high concentration of vitamin C), along with special enzymes that exist solely to protect sperm against oxidative damage.

When lifestyle factors such as toxin exposure or vitamin deficiencies cause too much oxidation or compromise the antioxidant defense system, the result is oxidative damage, which is thought to be a contributing factor in up to 80% of all cases of male infertility.[11]

Oxidation impacts the conventional semen parameters (sperm count, motility, and morphology) as well as the amount of damage to sperm DNA.[12] Research at the Cleveland Clinic has confirmed that men with high levels of oxidation in semen have more extensive DNA fragmentation and fewer normally functioning sperm.[13]

Medical problems such as infections, blockages, and enlarged veins (varicocele) account for about a quarter of cases of male infertility.[14] If you are affected by one of these conditions, you may need medication or a minor surgical procedure to improve your sperm quality. Yet such conventional medical treatment does not obviate the need to also pay attention to lifestyle and nutritional factors that can improve sperm quality.

The reality is that natural approaches to improving sperm quality may be even more critical in men with urological conditions because many conditions contribute to infertility by causing an increase in oxidative damage to sperm.[15]

Improving sperm quality may also be particularly critical when the female partner has poor egg quality. Unlike sperm, eggs have specialized machinery that can repair DNA damage, which allows eggs to overcome some of the negative effect of damaged sperm. Yet the DNA repair process only works effectively in good-quality eggs. An egg from an older woman may not be able to adequately repair the DNA damage from poor-quality sperm, making it even more difficult to conceive.[16]

The good news is that for most men, sperm quality is at least partly within your control through vitamin supplements and other simple steps you can take to guard against oxidative damage and thereby protect your fertility.

How to Improve Your Sperm Quality

Take a Daily Antioxidant Supplement

The single most important thing you can do to improve sperm quality is to take a daily supplement containing a combination of vitamins and antioxidants. Dozens of studies have clearly established that taking a daily antioxidant supplement improves sperm quality and increases the chance of conceiving.[17] This is true both for couples trying to conceive naturally and those undergoing fertility treatment.

One systematic review of the research in this area, analyzing 34 prior studies, determined that men who take antioxidant supplements had more than a 4 times higher chance of conceiving. There was also nearly a 5 times higher chance of a live birth when compared to men not taking antioxidants.[18] And no studies reported evidence of harmful side effects from the antioxidant therapy used.[19]

Some research suggests that antioxidants may be particularly powerful when infertility is caused by DNA damage within sperm. In one study, men with elevated DNA fragmentation were given vitamins C and E daily for two months following a failed attempt to achieve fertilization by ICSI (an approach similar to IVF, but sperm are injected directly into the eggs).[20] The researchers found an extraordinary improvement in the next attempt, with the clinical pregnancy rate jumping from 7% to 48%.

Different studies use different combinations of antioxidants, but the ones that have been studied the most in this context are vitamin C, vitamin E, zinc, folate, and selenium.[21] Vitamins C and E act directly as antioxidants, while zinc, folate, and selenium prevent oxidation in more complex ways, such as by assisting antioxidant enzymes. A deficiency in zinc or folate can also directly cause increased DNA damage.[22]

While many studies have tried to find out which of these vitamins (or which combination) help the most, you can cover all bases and probably get the most benefit by simply taking a daily multivitamin because all are found in standard multivitamins. A multivitamin designed specifically for men is a good option because it will probably contain more selenium. Ideally, you will start taking the vitamins two or three months before trying to conceive, but boosting your antioxidant levels for any time period before trying to conceive is likely to be beneficial.

If you want to go one step further, an additional antioxidant supplement to consider is CoQ10 — a vital antioxidant molecule found in just about every cell in the body. It is likely particularly important to sperm quality because it is not just an antioxidant but also a critical component of energy production.

Researchers have known for many years that there is a link between sperm quality and the level of CoQ10 naturally present in semen, with men having lower CoQ10 levels tending to show a lower sperm count and poor motility.[23]

In recent years, several different randomized, double-blind, placebo-controlled studies have determined that taking a CoQ10 supplement improves sperm concentration, motility, and morphology.[24] A recent study also found that the combination of CoQ10, antioxidants, and vitamin B12 not only improved traditional semen parameters but also significantly improved the integrity of DNA in sperm.[25]

One way in which CoQ10 is thought to improve sperm quality is by increasing the activity of antioxidant enzymes,[26] but it also likely has beneficial effects through enhanced energy production. Sufficient energy in the form of a molecule called ATP is absolutely critical for sperm production and motility. Cells can only make ATP when they have enough CoQ10. Although not yet proven, it is likely that CoQ10 supplements improve sperm quality by optimizing energy production.

If you choose to take CoQ10, the best form to take is known as ubiquinol (as explained in Chapter 6), and the usual recommended dose is 200 mg per day.[27]

Boost Your Antioxidant Levels Through Diet

To take full advantage of the power of antioxidants to boost sperm quality, it is a good idea to also maximize the antioxidants in your diet. This is borne out by years of scientific research finding that men with a diet higher in antioxidants are more likely to produce sperm with the correct number of chromosomes and tend to have improved semen parameters such as sperm count and motility.[28]

As just one example, a recent study found that men with higher fruit and cereal intake had better sperm quality.[29] One of the nutrients likely to be responsible for this benefit is folate, which is found in particularly large amounts in fruit, vegetables, and fortified cereal.

A little-known fact is that ensuring adequate folate intake is critical when trying to conceive for men, too — not just for women. While all women trying to conceive are told to take folate to prevent birth defects such as spina bifida, researchers now understand that folate is also imperative for men because it plays a critical role in protecting sperm DNA. In one study, men with a higher folate intake were less likely to produce sperm with the specific chromosomal error that causes Down syndrome.[30]

A recent study in California revealed that antioxidants may even prevent or reverse the increase in sperm DNA damage associated with aging. The study, which involved men having no known fertility problems, found that men with the highest total intake of vitamin C, vitamin E, zinc, and folate (from food and supplements) had much less sperm DNA damage.[31]

In fact, the men with the highest intake of these had sperm DNA quality similar to the younger men. This extraordinary finding suggests that we may be able to prevent a large part of the decline in fertility and increased risk of miscarriage and birth defects as men age.

A nutritious diet is important because it is likely that the specific antioxidants found in multivitamins are just a small percentage of the vast array of antioxidants found naturally in food. One additional antioxidant shown to be helpful for sperm quality but unlikely to be present in your typical multivitamin is lycopene.[32] This powerful antioxidant is found in tomatoes and becomes particularly concentrated once tomatoes are cooked, such as in tomato paste.

Other powerful antioxidants include anthocyanins, which give berries their dark purple color, and beta carotene, found in sweet potatoes and carrots. Additional well-known sources of antioxidants are green tea and dark chocolate, although little is known about how these antioxidants relate to sperm quality.

Until we know more about which antioxidants are most beneficial, the best approach is to eat a wide variety of fruits and vegetables, with a particular focus on the most brightly colored varieties, which are typically higher in antioxidants.

Reduce Your Exposure to Environmental Toxins

The power of lifestyle factors to influence sperm quality does not end with antioxidants. Everyday environmental toxins are thought to be a major contributing factor to the oxidative stress that is seen in up to 80% of infertile men. Toxins often cause increased oxidation by compromising the activity of antioxidant enzymes, along with a host of other harmful effects on sperm quality.

Over 80,000 chemicals are registered for use in the United States, yet only a small percentage have ever been analyzed for safety and even fewer for reproductive harm. Within the soup of chemicals we are all exposed to on a daily basis, it is not yet clear which toxins cause the most problems for men trying to conceive. However, so far the toxins with the clearest evidence of harm to sperm quality are the same ones shown to harm developing eggs: phthalates and BPA. They are both ubiquitous chemicals that have long been known to disrupt hormone activity (so called "endocrine disruptors").

Phthalates

Phthalates are a group of chemicals called "plasticizers" that are used in everything from cologne to laundry detergent to air freshener to soft, flexible plastic made from vinyl or PVC. As explained in more detail in Chapter 3, these chemicals are banned in children's toys, and some phthalates are banned in

227

personal care products in Europe, but overall very little has been done to curb the amount of phthalates we are exposed to on a daily basis. This is despite the fact that scientists have known for more than 20 years that these chemicals are absorbed into the body and interfere with critical hormones.

By acting as endocrine disruptors, phthalates cause a range of harmful effects, including genital malformations in baby boys exposed in utero. After many years of heated controversy, it now appears to be well established that phthalates also damage sperm in adult men.[33]

The concentration of phthalates that men are commonly exposed to has been shown to cause DNA damage in sperm while also reducing sperm quality by traditional measures. The damage may occur in a variety of ways, including altering hormone levels and causing oxidative stress. Specifically, higher phthalate levels have been linked to lower levels of testosterone and other hormones involved in male fertility.[34] A large study involving more than 10,000 people also revealed a link between higher levels of phthalates and more extensive oxidative stress throughout the body.[35]

Ultimately, even a small decline in sperm quality caused by phthalates may translate into a significant reduction in fertility. At the 2013 meeting of the American Society of Reproductive Medicine, researchers presented the results of a study investigating the relationship between phthalate levels and odds of conceiving in 500 couples. The researchers found that men who had the highest levels of phthalates in their bodies were 20% less likely to impregnate their partners over the course of a year.[36]

Men can reduce their exposure to phthalates by minimizing

the use of vinyl/PVC in the home, switching to shampoo, shaving cream, and deodorant labeled as "phthalate-free" (such as those made by Every Man Jack, Burt's Bees, and Caswell-Massey); avoiding unnecessary fragrance such as cologne and fragranced laundry detergent; and eating less processed food packaged in plastic.

BPA

Bisphenol A, or BPA for short, is another toxin that poses a potential danger to male fertility. It is commonly found in canned food, reusable plastic food storage containers, and the coating on paper receipts. Researchers have long been suspicious of BPA because it is an endocrine disruptor known to mimic the effects of estrogen.

In one of the earliest studies on the question of BPA and sperm quality, researchers at the University of Michigan found that higher urinary BPA levels were linked to lower sperm count, motility, and morphology, and a greater percentage of sperm DNA damage.[37]

Other studies have since confirmed that men with higher levels of BPA are more likely to have low sperm count and poor sperm quality.[38] In addition, animal studies have directly observed that exposure to BPA at levels equivalent to the amount humans are exposed to on a daily basis interferes with sperm production and causes DNA breakage in sperm.[39]

Even though some controversy still remains over the impact of BPA on sperm quality, there is now more than enough evidence to warrant caution. Luckily, it is easy to drastically reduce your exposure to BPA by only buying canned food labeled "BPA-free," using glass or stainless steel in the kitchen instead of plastic containers, and handling paper receipts as little as possible.

Lead and Other Heavy Metals

There is no question that lead poses a danger to human health. Fortunately, government action has significantly reduced lead in our environment. Even so, a little extra care is warranted if you are trying to conceive because researchers have found that men with higher lead levels tend to have a significantly lower sperm count and a greater percentage of abnormal sperm.[40]

A good way to reduce your exposure is to use a water filter certified to remove lead. For advice on specific brands, see the Environmental Working Group's online water filter buying guide.[41] Old paint is another source of possible lead exposure, so consider buying a test kit if your home has older, crumbling paint. Removing your shoes at the door is another good step to take because research has found that dirt tracked in from outside is the major source of lead in house dust.

Mercury is another heavy metal that could theoretically decrease male fertility, but at the time of writing there have only been isolated and inconsistent reports of mercury exposure impairing sperm quality.[42] Larger studies in the human population have shown no impact from higher mercury levels obtained through seafood consumption.[43] It may be the case that mercury remains more of a concern for women than men.

To manage some of the risk from the hundreds of other chemicals in the environment that could also contribute to poor sperm quality, you can err on the side of caution by minimizing exposure to chemicals known to have general toxic effects, such as pesticides, garden weed killer, and insect sprays. You should also exercise caution if you have a hobby or profession that involves welding or the use of pesticides or organic solvents such as formaldehyde. If you are particularly concerned about environmental toxins, the Environmental Working Group website has advice on how to avoid a dozen common endocrine disruptors, including fire retardants and arsenic (summarized at the end of Chapter 3).[44]

Chemicals in Commercial Lubricants

Research has recently revealed yet another group of chemicals that can interfere with fertility: those found in lubricants. Studies show that most lubricant brands significantly decrease sperm motility and increase DNA fragmentation.[45] The authors of one of these studies, published in 2014, noted that "commercial coital lubricants have been wrongly perceived to maintain fertility."[46] The only brand that does not show deleterious effects and can be considered "sperm-friendly" is Pre-seed, a product specifically designed for couples trying to conceive. Baby oil and canola oil also appear to leave sperm unharmed.

Cut Back on Alcohol

There is no doubt that heavy alcohol intake is associated with poor sperm quality,[47] but the evidence is much less consistent when it comes to the impact of moderate alcohol consumption. While many studies have shown no effect, some studies have reported a link between even moderate alcohol consumption by men and reduced fertility, particularly in the IVF context.

One study by researchers at the University of California evaluated whether male alcohol use during the in vitro fertilization program affected the reproductive outcome. The researchers found that the risk of not achieving a live birth more than doubled for men who drank one additional drink per day.[48] In this study, the effect on live birth rate appeared to be due in large part to an increased miscarriage rate for couples in which men drank alcohol in the month before the IVF cycle.

A more recent study in men attending a fertility clinic in Brazil found that alcohol consumption decreased sperm count, sperm motility, and fertilization rate.[49] Alcohol intake is known to increase oxidative stress throughout the body,[50] providing one explanation for how alcohol may negatively impact sperm.

While the occasional single glass of wine may have little effect, beyond this amount it may be worth exercising caution, particularly if you face an uphill battle trying to conceive.

Keep Your Distance from Cell Phones

Although commonly dismissed as a myth, scientific research actually does show that keeping a cell phone in your pocket could negatively impact sperm quality. Researchers at the Cleveland Clinic found that the use of cell phones decreases sperm count, motility, viability, and morphology, with a greater impact caused by a longer duration of daily exposure.[51] The same researchers also found that when sperm samples were exposed to radiation from a cell phone for one hour, there was a significant decrease in sperm motility and viability, and an increase in signs of oxidation.[52]

The radiofrequency electromagnetic waves emitted by cell phones are thought to damage sperm through a combination of heat generated by the electromagnetic waves and other effects, likely including oxidative stress.[53] These effects all depend on the cell phone being in very close physical proximity, so you can decrease your exposure by keeping your cell phone out of your pocket whenever possible.

Stay Cool

Researchers have known for more than 40 years that elevated temperatures impair sperm quality. The impact of heat on sperm quality is readily apparent from the effect of a fever, which causes a drop in sperm count and motility.[54] The longer the fever, the worse the impact on sperm quality.

Other factors also increase temperature where it matters: sitting all day, taking hot baths or showers, and wearing tight-fitting underwear.[55] In one 6-month study, researchers witnessed a 50% decrease in sperm parameters in men wearing tight-fitting underwear. Sperm parameters improved after subjects switched to loose-fitting underwear.[56]

Many fertility clinics advise men to avoid hot baths and showers in the week before sperm sample collection, but we know there are other ways to avoid overheating, such as taking regular breaks from sitting and wearing loose-fitting underwear. We also know that a week could be too short. The full process of sperm production takes over two months, and it is likely that early stages of sperm production are just as vulnerable to heat. The longer you can keep things cool, the better.

Action Plan for Sperm Quality

- Take a daily multivitamin, ideally several months before trying to conceive, and consider also taking a CoQ10 supplement.

- Further boost your vitamin and antioxidant levels with a diet rich in brightly colored fruits and vegetables.

- Take steps to reduce your exposure to toxins known to damage sperm: phthalates, BPA, lead, and the chemicals in commercial lubricants.

- Reduce alcohol consumption, particularly in the lead-up to IVF.

- Keep your cell phone out of your pocket when you can.

- Stay cool where it counts.

CHAPTER 13

Putting It All Together: Your Complete Action Plan

"Forget past mistakes. Forget failures. Forget everything except what you're going to do now and do it."
— WILLIAM DURANT

The Basic Plan

WHETHER YOU ARE just starting to think about getting pregnant and have no reason to expect any difficulty or you have been struggling with infertility for several years, all women trying to conceive can benefit from the basic steps that have been shown to improve egg quality and fertility. To increase your chance of conceiving and reduce the risk of miscarriage:

- Start taking a daily prenatal multivitamin as soon as possible, ideally at least three months before trying to conceive. Doing so may not only prevent serious birth defects but will also protect your eggs and may therefore help you conceive sooner. A brand that includes 800 mcg of folic acid rather than 400 mcg may offer additional benefit. If you have a sensitive stomach, try several brands until you find one that works and take the supplement before bed. Good-quality brands include Rainbow Light and New Chapter Organics.

- Consider adding a daily CoQ10 supplement to enhance energy production inside developing eggs and possibly prevent chromosomal errors. The most effective form of CoQ10 is ubiquinol, and the basic dose is 100 mg, preferably taken in the morning with food.

- Reduce your exposure to the hormone-disrupting toxin BPA by only buying canned food labeled "BPA-free," replacing plastic food storage containers with glass, and handling paper receipts as little as possible.

- Minimize exposure to phthalates by avoiding nail polish and perfume, and by switching to fragrance-free or phthalate-free skin-care, hair-care, laundry, and cleaning products, such as those made by The Honest Company, Alterna, Neutrogena Naturals, California Baby, and Seventh Generation.

- Further reduce your phthalate exposure by watching out for soft, flexible plastic products made of vinyl or PVC. Replace these items with safer alternatives made out of fabric instead of plastic, or specifically labeled as "phthalate-free" or "PVC-free."

- Reduce sugar and refined carbohydrates in your diet and shift toward a Mediterranean diet based on fruits, vegetables, minimally processed grains, olive oil, nuts, and lean protein.

Intermediate Plan: Difficulty Conceiving

If you are having trouble getting pregnant but have not yet been diagnosed with any specific fertility problems, there are some further steps that may help you conceive sooner. In addition to following the advice listed above for the basic plan:

- Ask your doctor to test you for vitamin D deficiency, celiac disease, and underactive thyroid. These three conditions often contribute to unexplained infertility and are typically overlooked by fertility specialists. They are also easy to treat.

- Consider taking a higher dose of CoQ10 (ubiquinol), such as 200 mg, and taking one or more additional antioxidant such as vitamin E (200 IU), vitamin C (500 mg), or alpha-lipoic acid (in the form of R-alpha-lipoic acid, 100 mg to 600 mg per day on an empty stomach). Studies have shown that women with unexplained infertility often have compromised antioxidant defenses in their ovarian follicles and that antioxidant supplements can reduce the time it takes them to conceive.

Intermediate Plan: Polycystic Ovary Syndrome or Irregular Ovulation

PCOS is one of the most common causes of infertility. Symptoms include weight gain, acne, facial hair, and irregular menstrual cycles or cycles longer than 35 days. PCOS causes infertility by disturbing normal ovulation and reducing egg quality. In addition to the steps listed above for the basic plan, to improve egg quality and rebalance hormones:

- Consider taking a myo-inositol supplement for two or three months before trying to conceive. The typical recommended dose is 4 g per day, divided into two doses: half in the morning and half at night.

- Be particularly vigilant about minimizing your exposure to BPA. Studies have found that BPA levels are often significantly higher in women with PCOS, and BPA appears to contribute to the hormonal imbalances that are characteristic of PCOS.

- Prevent spikes in blood sugar and insulin levels by strictly limiting sugar and refined carbohydrates in your diet. Insulin raises testosterone levels, which is often a major contributor to infertility in PCOS.

- Consider also taking an alpha-lipoic acid supplement to control the oxidative stress that contributes to poor egg quality in PCOS. The dose shown to improve fertility in women with PCOS is 600 mg, twice per day.

Advanced Plan: Recurrent Miscarriage

While there are various medical causes of recurrent miscarriage, including blood clotting and immune disorders, nearly half of all early miscarriages are caused by chromosomal errors in the egg. By improving your egg quality, you may be able to reduce the chance of chromosomal errors occurring and thereby reduce your risk of miscarriage. In addition to the steps listed above for the basic plan:

- Take a daily CoQ10 (ubiquinol) supplement of up to 300 mg to enhance energy production in developing eggs and encourage correct chromosome processing. You may also want to consider taking one or more additional antioxidants such as vitamin E (200 IU), vitamin C (500 mg), or alpha-lipoic acid (in the form of R-alpha-lipoic acid, 100 mg to 600 mg per day on an empty stomach).

- Consider taking a myo-inositol supplement if you have insulin resistance, irregular ovulation, or other symptoms of polycystic ovarian syndrome (4 g per day, divided in 2 doses). Insulin resistance is much more common in women with a history of multiple miscarriages, and myo-inositol may be able to address this problem.

- Ask your doctor whether you need a higher dose of folic acid, such as 4000 mcg per day.

- Ask your doctor to test you for underactive thyroid, a major cause of recurrent miscarriage. If you are diagnosed with hypothyroidism, insist on proper treatment before trying to conceive again. Studies have found that in women with autoimmune thyroid disease, treatment with an added thyroid hormone called levothyroxin reduces the miscarriage rate by more than 50%.

- Ask your doctor to test you for celiac disease, which dramatically increases miscarriage risk. If you have celiac disease, closely follow a gluten-free diet to prevent the immune reactions and vitamin deficiencies that increase the chance of losing a pregnancy.

- To further prevent the chromosomal errors that cause many miscarriages, consider taking DHEA if you are trying to conceive through IVF and have diminished ovarian reserve.

- Make sure your male partner is also taking a daily multivitamin and has a diet rich in anti-oxidants, particularly if he is over the age of 40. Also ask your partner to strictly limit his alcohol consumption.

Advanced Plan: Trying to Conceive Through IVF with Diminished Ovarian Reserve:

If you have been diagnosed with diminished ovarian reserve or age-related infertility, you have the most to gain from an aggressive plan to improve egg quality. In addition to the steps listed above for the basic plan:

- You may benefit from a higher-dose of CoQ10 (ubiquinol), such as 300 mg. You may also want to take one or more additional antioxidants in the form of vitamin E (200 IU), vitamin C (500 mg) or alpha-lipoic acid (as R-alpha-lipoic acid, 100 mg to 600 mg per day on an empty stomach) for three months before your next IVF cycle.

- To increase your egg numbers and prevent chromosomal errors in eggs, consider also taking a DHEA supplement for three months before your next IVF cycle. The formulation of DHEA is particularly important because if not formulated correctly, it will not be absorbed. Look for a brand that is pharmaceutical grade, micronized, and potency guaranteed, such as Fertinatal. The typical dose is 25 mg, three times per day.

- To further boost egg quality, consider taking a melatonin supplement at the start of your next IVF cycle, when you begin injectable medications. The typical dose is a 3 mg tablet shortly before bed. If side effects bother you, take a smaller dose.

- Ask your doctor to test you for underactive thyroid, a common cause of diminished ovarian reserve in younger women.

- Carefully limit sugar and refined carbohydrates in your diet and maximize vitamins and antioxidants.

- Make sure your male partner is also taking a daily multivitamin and has a diet rich in antioxidants.

Author's Note

EGG QUALITY HAS such profound implications for fertility and miscarriage risk that all women who are trying to conceive deserve to know what they can do to protect their own egg quality. If you found this book useful please help spread the word to other women who are struggling with infertility.

My hope is that the information provided in this book will allow others to overcome fertility challenges caused by poor egg quality and finally realize their dream of having a healthy baby. In short, I hope that others can be as fortunate as I have been. My own success story is pictured on the back cover of this book: my beautiful baby boy at ten days old.

Notes

Scientific publications are available from
the National Institutes of Health database
at www.ncbi.nlm.nih.gov/pubmed

Introduction

1 Ehrlich S, Williams PL, Missmer SA, Flaws JA, Ye X, Calafat AM, Petrozza JC, Wright D, Hauser R. Urinary bisphenol A concentrations and early reproductive health outcomes among women undergoing IVF. Hum Reprod. 2012 Dec;27(12):3583-92.

2 Wright VC, Chang J, Jeng G, Macaluso M. Assisted reproductive technology surveillance—United States, 2003. MMWR Surveill Summ. 2006 May 26;55(4):1-22.

3 Stagnaro-Green A.Thyroid antibodies and miscarriage: where are we at a generation later? J Thyroid Res. 2011;2011:841949.

4 Thangaratinam S, Tan A, Knox E, Kilby MD, Franklyn J, Coomarasamy A. Association between thyroid autoantibodies and miscarriage and preterm birth: meta-analysis of evidence. BMJ. 2011 May 9;342:d2616.

5 Sugiura-Ogasawara M, Ozaki Y, Katano K, Suzumori N, Kitaori T, Mizutani E. Abnormal embryonic karyotype is the most frequent cause of recurrent miscarriage. Hum Reprod. 2012 Aug;27(8):2297-303 ("Suguira-Ogasawara 2012").

6 Macklon NS, Geraedts JP, Fauser BC. Conception to ongoing pregnancy: the 'black box' of early pregnancy loss. Hum Reprod Update. 2002 Jul-Aug;8(4):333-43 ("Macklon 2002").

Chapter 1: Understanding Egg Quality

1 Sugiura-Ogasawara M, Ozaki Y, Katano K, Suzumori N, Kitaori T, Mizutani E. Abnormal embryonic karyotype is the most frequent cause of recurrent miscarriage. Hum Reprod. 2012 Aug;27(8):2297-303;

Macklon NS, Geraedts JP, Fauser BC. Conception to ongoing pregnancy: the 'black box' of early pregnancy loss. Hum Reprod Update. 2002 Jul-Aug;8(4):333-43

2 Macklon 2002.

3 Hassold T, Hall H, Hunt P. The origin of human aneuploidy: where we have been, where we are going. Hum Mol Genet. 2007;16(Spec No. 2):R203–R208. ("Hassold and Hunt 2007"); Macklon 2002; Sher G, Keskintepe L, Keskintepe M, Ginsburg M, Maassarani G, Yakut T, Baltaci V, Kotze D, Unsal E.Oocyte karyotyping by comparative genomic hybridization provides a highly reliable method for selecting "competent" embryos, markedly improving in vitro fertilization outcome: a multiphase study. Fertil Steril. 2007 May;87(5):1033-40.

4 Fragouli E, Alfarawati S, Goodall NN, Sánchez-García JF, Colls P, Wells D. The cytogenetics of polar bodies: insights into female meiosis and the diagnosis of aneuploidy. Mol Hum Reprod. 2011 May;17(5):286-95. ("Fragouli 2011").

5 van den Berg MM, van Maarle MC, van Wely M, Goddijn M. Genetics of early miscarriage. Biochim Biophys Acta. 2012 Dec;1822(12):1951-9; ("van den Berg 2012").
Macklon 2002

6 Macklon 2002.

7 Suguira-Ogasawara 2012.

8 Kushnir VA, Frattarelli JL. Aneuploidy in abortuses following IVF and ICSI. J Assist Reprod Genet. 2009 Mar;26(2-3):93-7;
Kim JW, Lee WS, Yoon TK, Seok HH, Cho JH, Kim YS, Lyu SW, Shim SH. Chromosomal abnormalities in spontaneous abortion after assisted reproductive treatment. BMC Med Genet. 2010 Nov 3;11:153;
van den Berg 2012

9 Macklon 2002.

10 Allen EG, Freeman SB, Druschel C, Hobbs CA, O'Leary LA, Romitti PA, Royle MH, Torfs CP, Sherman SL. Maternal age and risk for trisomy 21 assessed by the origin of chromosome nondisjunction: a report from the Atlanta and National Down Syndrome Projects. Hum Genet. 2009 Feb;125(1):41-52.

11 Fragouli 2011; Macklon 2002.

12 Pellestor F, Andréo B, Anahory T, Hamamah S. The occurrence of aneuploidy in human: lessons from the cytogenetic studies of human oocytes. Eur J Med Genet. 2006 Mar-Apr;49(2):103-16; Fragouli 2011; Macklon 2002.

13 Kuliev A, Zlatopolsky Z, Kirillova I, Spivakova J, Cieslak Janzen J. Meiosis errors in over 20,000 oocytes studied in the practice of preimplantation aneuploidy testing. Reprod Biomed Online. 2011 Jan;22(1):2-8.

14 Fragouli 2011.

15 Fragouli 2011.

16 http://www.colocrm.com/AboutCCRM/SuccessRates/2011statistics. aspx

17 Schoolcraft WB, Fragouli E, Stevens J, Munne S, Katz-Jaffe MG, Wells D. Clinical application of comprehensive chromosomal screening at the blastocyst stage. Fertil Steril. 2010 Oct;94(5):1700-6.

18 Katz-Jaffe MG, Surrey ES, Minjarez DA, Gustofson RL, Stevens JM, Schoolcraft WB. Association of abnormal ovarian reserve parameters with a higher incidence of aneuploid blastocysts. Obstet Gynecol. 2013 Jan;121(1):71-7.

19 Yang Z, Liu J, Collins GS, Salem SA, Liu X, Lyle SS, Peck AC, Sills ES, Salem RD. Selection of single blastocysts for fresh transfer via standard morphology assessment alone and with array CGH for good prognosis IVF patients: results from a randomized pilot study. Mol Cytogenet. 2012 May 2;5(1):24.

20 Munné S, Held KR, Magli CM, Ata B, Wells D, Fragouli E, Baukloh V, Fischer R, Gianaroli L. Intra-age, intercenter, and intercycle differences in chromosome abnormalities in oocytes. Fertil Steril. 2012 Apr;97(4):935-42.

21 Hassold T, Hunt P. Maternal age and chromosomally abnormal pregnancies: what we know and what we wish we knew. Curr Opin Pediatr. 2009 Dec;21(6):703-8.

22 Nagaoka SI, Hassold TJ, Hunt PA. Human aneuploidy: mechanisms and new insights into an age-old problem. Nat Rev Genet. 2012 Jun 18;13(7):493-504; Fragouli 2011;

23 Bentov Y, Yavorska T, Esfandiari N, Jurisicova A, Casper RF. The contribution of mitochondrial function to reproductive aging. J Assist Reprod Genet. 2011 Sep;28(9):773-83.

24 Van Blerkom J. Mitochondrial function in the human oocyte and embryo and their role in developmental competence. Mitochondrion. 2011 Sep;11(5):797-813. ("Van Blerkom 2011").

25 Van Blerkom 2011.

26 Shigenaga MK, Hagen TM, Ames BN. Oxidative damage and mitochondrial decay in aging. Proc Natl Acad Sci USA. 1994 91:10771–8.

27 Eichenlaub-Ritter U, Wieczorek M, Lüke S, Seidel T. Age related changes in mitochondrial function and new approaches to study redox regulation in mammalian oocytes in response to age or maturation conditions. Mitochondrion. 2011 Sep;11(5):783-96; Van Blerkom 2011.

28 Interview with Dr. Robert Casper, published in The Spectator, 11/19/2011. http://www.spectator.co.uk/features/7396723/resetting-the-clock/

Chapter 2: The Dangers of BPA

1 Dr. Patricia Hunt, personal communication. 2/6/2014.

2 Hunt PA, Koehler KE, Susiarjo M, Hodges CA, Ilagan A, Voigt RC, Thomas S, Thomas BF, Hassold TJ. Bisphenol a exposure causes meiotic aneuploidy in the female mouse. Curr Biol. 2003 Apr 1;13(7):546-53. ("Hunt 2003").

3 Dr. Patricia Hunt, personal communication. 2/6/2014.

4 Hunt 2003.

5 vom Saal FS, Akingbemi BT, Belcher SM, Birnbaum LS, Crain DA, Eriksen M, Farabollini F, Guillette LJ Jr, Hauser R, Heindel JJ, Ho SM, Hunt PA, Iguchi T, Jobling S, Kanno J, Keri RA, Knudsen KE, Laufer H, LeBlanc GA, Marcus M, McLachlan JA, Myers JP, Nadal A, Newbold RR, Olea N, Prins GS, Richter CA, Rubin BS, Sonnenschein C, Soto AM, Talsness CE, Vandenbergh JG, Vandenberg LN, Walser-Kuntz DR, Watson CS, Welshons WV, Wetherill Y, Zoeller RT. Chapel Hill bisphenol A expert panel consensus statement: integration of mechanisms, effects in animals and potential to impact human health at current levels of exposure. Reprod Toxicol. 2007 Aug-Sep;24(2):131-8. ("vom Saal 2007").

6 Lang IA, Galloway TS, Scarlett A, Henley WE, Depledge M, Wallace RB, Melzer D. Association of urinary bisphenol A concentration with medical disorders and laboratory abnormalities in adults. JAMA. 2008 Sep 17;300(11):1303-10; Shankar A, Teppala S. Relationship between urinary bisphenol A levels and diabetes mellitus. J Clin Endocrinol Metab. 2011 Dec; 96(12):3822-6; Silver MK, O'Neill MS, Sowers MR, Park SK. Urinary bisphenol A and type-2 diabetes in U.S. adults: data from NHANES 2003-2008. PLoS One. 2011;6(10):e26868.

7 Melzer D, Rice NE, Lewis C, Henley WE, Galloway TS. Association of urinary bisphenol a concentration with heart disease: evidence from NHANES 2003/06. PLoS One. 2010 Jan 13;5(1):e8673.

8 Calafat AM, Ye X, Wong LY, Reidy JA, Needham LL. Exposure of the U.S. population to bisphenol A and 4-tertiary-octylphenol: 2003-2004. Environ Health Perspect. 2008 Jan;116(1):39-44.

9 Stahlhut RW, Welshons WV, Swan SH. Bisphenol A data in NHANES suggest longer than expected half-life, substantial nonfood exposure, or both. Environ Health Perspect. 2009 May;117(5):784-9.
Vandenberg LN, Chahoud I, Heindel JJ, Padmanabhan V, Paumgartten FJ, Schoenfelder G. Urinary, circulating, and tissue biomonitoring studies indicate widespread exposure to bisphenol A. Environ Health Perspect. 2010 Aug;118(8):1055-70.

10 Kitamura S, Suzuki T, Sanoh S, Kohta R, Jinno N, Sugihara K, Yoshihara S, Fujimoto N, Watanabe H, Ohta S. Comparative study of the endocrine-disrupting activity of bisphenol A and 19 related compounds. Toxicol Sci. 2005 Apr;84(2):249-59;
Welshons WV, Nagel SC, vom Saal FS. Large effects from small exposures. III. Endocrine mechanisms mediating effects of bisphenol A at levels of human exposure. Endocrinology. 2006 Jun;147(6 Suppl):S56-69. ("Welshons 2006").

11 Kuiper GG, Lemmen JG, Carlsson B, Corton JC, Safe SH, van der Saag PT, van der Burg B, Gustafsson JA. Interaction of estrogenic chemicals and phytoestrogens with estrogen receptor beta. Endocrinology. 1998 Oct;139(10):4252-63.

12 Wozniak AL, Bulayeva NN, Watson CS. Xenoestrogens at picomolar to nanomolar concentrations trigger membrane estrogen receptor-alpha-mediated Ca2+ fluxes and prolactin release in GH3/B6 pituitary tumor cells. Environ Health Perspect. 2005 Apr;113(4):431-9;
Welshons 2006.

13 Sabrina Tavernise, F.D.A. Makes It Official: BPA Can't Be Used in Baby Bottles and Cups NYTimes, July 17, 2012.

14 http://www.commondreams.org/headline/2012/07/17-4

15 March 2012 Consumer Update. [http://www.fda.gov/ForConsumers/ConsumerUpdates/ucm297954

16 Vandenberg LN, Maffini MV, Sonnenschein C, Rubin BS, Soto AM. Bisphenol-A and the great divide: a review of controversies in the field of endocrine disruption. Endocr Rev. 2009 Feb;30(1):75-95. ("Vandenberg 2009").

17 Tyl RW, Myers CB, Marr MC, Thomas BF, Keimowitz AR, Brine DR, Veselica MM, Fail PA, Chang TY, Seely JC, Joiner RL, Butala JH, Dimond SS, Cagen SZ, Shiotsuka RN, Stropp GD, Waechter JM. Three-generation reproductive toxicity study of

dietary bisphenol A in CD Sprague-Dawley rats. Toxicol Sci. 2002 Jul;68(1):121-46; ("Tyl 2002").

Tyl RW, Myers CB, Marr MC, Sloan CS, Castillo NP, Veselica MM, Seely JC, Dimond SS, Van Miller JP, Shiotsuka RN, Beyer D, Hentges SG, Waechter JM Jr. Two-generation reproductive toxicity study of dietary bisphenol A in CD-1 (Swiss) mice. Toxicol Sci. 2008 Aug;104(2):362-84. ("Tyl 2008").

18 Myers JP, vom Saal FS, Akingbemi BT, Arizono K, Belcher S, Colborn T, Chahoud I, Crain DA, Farabollini F, Guillette LJ Jr, Hassold T, Ho SM, Hunt PA, Iguchi T, Jobling S, Kanno J, Laufer H, Marcus M, McLachlan JA, Nadal A, Oehlmann J, Olea N, Palanza P, Parmigiani S, Rubin BS, Schoenfelder G, Sonnenschein C, Soto AM, Talsness CE, Taylor JA, Vandenberg LN, Vandenbergh JG, Vogel S, Watson CS, Welshons WV, Zoeller RT. Why public health agencies cannot depend on good laboratory practices as a criterion for selecting data: the case of bisphenol A. Environ Health Perspect. 2009 Mar;117(3):309-15.

19 Tyl 2002; http://www.factsaboutbpa.org/about-us]

20 vom Saal FS, Nagel SC, Timms BG, Welshons WV. Implications for human health of the extensive bisphenol A literature showing adverse effects at low doses: a response to attempts to mislead the public. Toxicology. 2005 Sep 1;212(2-3):244-52;
vom Saal FS, Akingbemi BT, Belcher SM, Crain DA, Crews D, Guidice LC, Hunt PA, Leranth C, Myers JP, Nadal A, Olea N, Padmanabhan V, Rosenfeld CS, Schneyer A, Schoenfelder G, Sonnenschein C, Soto AM, Stahlhut RW, Swan SH, Vandenberg LN, Wang HS, Watson CS, Welshons WV, Zoeller RT. Flawed experimental design reveals the need for guidelines requiring appropriate positive controls in endocrine disruption research. Toxicol Sci. 2010 Jun;115(2):612-3;

21 vom Saal FS, Hughes C. An extensive new literature concerning low-dose effects of bisphenol A shows the need for a new risk assessment. Environ Health Perspect. 2005 Aug;113(8):926-33.

22 FDA Science Board Subcommittee on Bisphenol A, Scientific Peer-Review of the Draft Assessment of Bisphenol A for Use in Food Contact Applications, October 31, 2008.

23 Lamb, J. D., M. S. Bloom, F. S. Vom Saal, J. A. Taylor, J. R. Sandler, and V. Y. Fujimoto. "Serum Bisphenol A (BPA) and reproductive outcomes in couples undergoing IVF." Fertil Steril. 2008; 90: S186.

24 Fujimoto VY, Kim D, vom Saal FS, Lamb JD, Taylor JA, Bloom MS. Serum unconjugated bisphenol A concentrations in women

may adversely influence oocyte quality during in vitro fertilization. Fertil Steril. 2011 Apr;95(5):1816-9.

25 Mok-Lin E, Ehrlich S, Williams PL, Petrozza J, Wright DL, Calafat AM, Ye X, Hauser R. Urinary bisphenol A concentrations and ovarian response among women undergoing IVF. Int J Androl. 2010 Apr;33(2):385-93. ("Mok-Lin 2010").

26 Ehrlich S, Williams PL, Missmer SA, Flaws JA, Ye X, Calafat AM, Petrozza JC, Wright D, Hauser R. Urinary bisphenol A concentrations and early reproductive health outcomes among women undergoing IVF. Hum Reprod. 2012 Dec;27(12):3583-92

27 Ehrlich S, Williams PL, Missmer SA, Flaws JA, Berry KF, Calafat AM, Ye X, Petrozza JC, Wright D, Hauser R. Urinary bisphenol A concentrations and implantation failure among women undergoing in vitro fertilization. Environ Health Perspect. 2012 Jul;120(7):978-83.

28 Berger RG, Foster WG, deCatanzaro D. Bisphenol-A exposure during the period of blastocyst implantation alters uterine morphology and perturbs measures of estrogen and progesterone receptor expression in mice. Reprod Toxicol. 2010 Nov;30(3):393-400;
Xiao S, Diao H, Smith MA, Song X, Ye X. Preimplantation exposure to bisphenol A (BPA) affects embryo transport, preimplantation embryo development, and uterine receptivity in mice. Reprod Toxicol. 2011 Dec;32(4):434-41;

29 Sugiura-Ogasawara M, Ozaki Y, Sonta S, Makino T, Suzumori K. Exposure to bisphenol A is associated with recurrent miscarriage. Hum Reprod. 2005 Aug;20(8):2325-9.

30 R.B. Lathi et al, Maternal Serum Bisphenol-A (BPA) Level Is Positively Associated with Miscarriage Risk, O-6 , 69th Annual Meeting of the American Society for Reproductive Medicine, October 14, 2013.

31 Can A, Semiz O, Cinar O. Bisphenol-A induces cell cycle delay and alters centrosome and spindle microtubular organization in oocytes during meiosis. Mol Hum Reprod. 2005 Jun;11(6):389-96. ("Can 2005").

32 Lenie S, Cortvrindt R, Eichenlaub-Ritter U, Smitz J.Continuous exposure to bisphenol A during in vitro follicular development induces meiotic abnormalities. Mutat Res. 2008 Mar 12;651(1-2):71-81.

33 Xu J, Osuga Y, Yano T, Morita Y, Tang X, Fujiwara T, Takai Y, Matsumi H, Koga K, Taketani Y, Tsutsumi O. Bisphenol A induces apoptosis and G2-to-M arrest of ovarian granulosa cells. Biochem Biophys Res Commun. 2002 Mar 29;292(2):456-62.
Brieño-Enríquez MA, Robles P, Camats-Tarruella N, García-Cruz R, Roig I, Cabero L, Martínez F, Caldés MG. Human

meiotic progression and recombination are affected by Bisphenol A exposure during in vitro human oocyte development. Hum Reprod. 2011 Oct;26(10):2807-18.

34 Lee SG, Kim JY, Chung JY, Kim YJ, Park JE, Oh S, Yoon YD, Yoo KS, Yoo YH, Kim JM. Bisphenol A exposure during adulthood causes augmentation of follicular atresia and luteal regression by decreasing 17β-estradiol synthesis via downregulation of aromatase in rat ovary. Environ Health Perspect. 2013 Jun;121(6):663-9.

35 Grasselli F, Baratta L, Baioni L, Bussolati S, Ramoni R, Grolli S, Basini G. Bisphenol A disrupts granulosa cell function. Domest Anim Endocrinol. 2010 Jul;39(1):34-9;
Zhou W, Liu J, Liao L, Han S, Liu J. Effect of bisphenol A on steroid hormone production in rat ovarian theca-interstitial and granulosa cells. Mol Cell Endocrinol. 2008 Feb 13;283(1-2):12-8; Pertez 2011.

36 Mok-Lin 2010

37 Moriyama K, Tagami T, Akamizu T, Usui T, Saijo M, Kanamoto N, et al. Thyroid hormone action is disrupted by bisphenol A as an antagonist. J Clin Endocrinol Metab. 2002;87:5185–5190.
Meeker JD, Calafat AM, Hauser R. Urinary bisphenol A concentrations in relation to serum thyroid and reproductive hormone levels in men from an infertility clinic. Environ Sci Technol. 2010;44:1458–1463.
Soriano S, Alonso-Magdalena P, García-Arévalo M, Novials A, Muhammed SJ, Salehi A, Gustafsson JA, Quesada I, Nadal A. Rapid insulinotropic action of low doses of bisphenol-A on mouse and human islets of Langerhans: role of estrogen receptor β. PLoS One. 2012;7(2):e31109.;
Ropero AB, Alonso-Magdalena P, García-García E, Ripoll C, Fuentes E, Nadal A. Bisphenol-A disruption of the endocrine pancreas and blood glucose homeostasis. Int J Androl. 2008 Apr;31(2):194-200.

38 Peretz J, Gupta RK, Singh J, Hernández-Ochoa I, Flaws JA. Bisphenol A impairs follicle growth, inhibits steroidogenesis, and downregulates rate-limiting enzymes in the estradiol biosynthesis pathway. Toxicol Sci. 2011 Jan;119(1):209-17. ("Peretz 2011").
Lee SG, Kim JY, Chung JY, Kim YJ, Park JE, Oh S, Yoon YD, Yoo KS, Yoo YH, Kim JM. Bisphenol A exposure during adulthood causes augmentation of follicular atresia and luteal regression by decreasing 17β-estradiol synthesis via downregulation of aromatase in rat ovary. Environ Health Perspect. 2013 Jun;121(6):663-9.

39 Wang Q, Moley KH. Maternal diabetes and oocyte quality. Mitochondrion. 2010 Aug;10(5):403-10; Rajani S, Chattopadhyay R, Goswami SK, Ghosh S, Sharma S, Chakravarty B. Assessment of oocyte quality in polycystic ovarian syndrome and endometriosis by spindle imaging and reactive oxygen species levels in follicular fluid and its relationship with IVF-ET outcome. J Hum Reprod Sci. 2012 May;5(2):187-93.

40 Takeuchi T, Tsutsumi O, Ikezuki Y, Takai Y, Taketani Y. Positive relationship between androgen and the endocrine disruptor, bisphenol A, in normal women and women with ovarian dysfunction. Endocr J. 2004 Apr;51(2):165-9.

Kandaraki, Eleni, Antonis Chatzigeorgiou, Sarantis Livadas, Eleni Palioura, Frangiscos Economou, Michael Koutsilieris, Sotiria Palimeri, Dimitrios Panidis, and Evanthia Diamanti-Kandarakis. "Endocrine disruptors and polycystic ovary syndrome (PCOS): elevated serum levels of bisphenol A in women with PCOS." Journal of Clinical Endocrinology & Metabolism 96, no. 3 (2011): E480-E484.

41 Shankar 2011;Silver 2011.

42 Soriano S, Alonso-Magdalena P, García-Arévalo M, Novials A, Muhammed SJ, Salehi A, Gustafsson JA, Quesada I, Nadal A. Rapid insulinotropic action of low doses of bisphenol-A on mouse and human islets of Langerhans: role of estrogen receptor β. PLoS One. 2012;7(2):e31109;

Ropero AB, Alonso-Magdalena P, García-García E, Ripoll C, Fuentes E, Nadal A. Bisphenol-A disruption of the endocrine pancreas and blood glucose homeostasis. Int J Androl. 2008 Apr;31(2):194-200

43 Masuno H, Kidani T, Sekiya K, Sakayama K, Shiosaka T, Yamamoto H, Honda K. Bisphenol A in combination with insulin can accelerate the conversion of 3T3-L1 fibroblasts to adipocytes. J Lipid Res. 2002 May;43(5):676-84.

Hugo ER, Brandebourg TD, Woo JG, Loftus J, Alexander JW, Ben-Jonathan N. Bisphenol A at environmentally relevant doses inhibits adiponectin release from human adipose tissue explants and adipocytes. Environ Health Perspect. 2008 Dec;116(12):1642-7.

44 Rudel RA, Gray JM, Engel CL, Rawsthorne TW, Dodson RE, Ackerman JM, Rizzo J, Nudelman JL, Brody JG. Food packaging and bisphenol A and bis(2-ethylhexyl) phthalate exposure: findings from a dietary intervention. Environ Health Perspect. 2011 Jul;119(7):914-20.

45 Brede C, Fjeldal P, Skjevrak I, Herikstad H. Increased migration levels of bisphenol A from polycarbonate baby bottles after dishwashing, boiling and brushing. Food Addit Contam. 2003 Jul;20(7):684-9.

46 Yang CZ, Yaniger SI, Jordan VC, Klein DJ, Bittner GD. Most plastic products release estrogenic chemicals: a potential health problem that can be solved. Environ Health Perspect. 2011;119:989–96.

47 Lakind JS, Naiman DQ. Daily intake of bisphenol A and potential sources of exposure: 2005-2006 National Health and Nutrition Examination Survey. J Expo Sci Environ Epidemiol. 2011 May-Jun;21(3):272-9.

48 Kang JH, Kondo F. Bisphenol A migration from cans containing coffee and caffeine. Food Addit Contam. 2002 Sep;19(9):886-90; J.A. Brotons, et al., Xenoestrogens released from lacquer coatings in food cans, Health Prespect.103 (1995) 608-612; Howdeshell KL, Peterman PH, Judy BM, Taylor JA, Orazio CE, Ruhlen RL, Vom Saal FS, Welshons WV. Bisphenol A is released from used polycarbonate animal cages into water at room temperature. Environ Health Perspect. 2003 Jul;111(9):1180-7.

49 Bae B, Jeong JH, Lee SJ. The quantification and characterization of endocrine disruptor bisphenol-A leaching from epoxy resin. Water Sci Technol. 2002;46(11-12):381-7.

50 Carwile J. L. et al, Canned Soup Consumption and Urinary Bisphenol A: A Randomized Crossover Trial. JAMA 306: 20 (2011): 2218-2219.

51 Geens T, Goeyens L, Covaci A. Are potential sources for human exposure to bisphenol-A overlooked? Int J Hyg Environ Health. 2011 Sep;214(5):339-47.

52 Biedermann S, Tschudin P, Grob K. Transfer of bisphenol A from thermal printer paper to the skin. Anal Bioanal Chem. 2010 Sep;398(1):571-6. Zalko D, Jacques C, Duplan H, Bruel S, Perdu E.Viable skin efficiently absorbs and metabolizes bisphenol A.Chemosphere. 2011 Jan;82(3):424-30.

53 Lunder 2010, "BPA Coats Cash Register Receipts", http://www.ewg.org/bpa-in-store-receipts

54 vom Saal 2007.

55 Takahashi O, Oishi S. Disposition of orally administered 2,2-Bis(4-hydroxyphenyl)propane (Bisphenol A) in pregnant rats and the placental transfer to fetuses. Environ Health Perspect. 2000 Oct;108(10):931-5; Vom saal 2007.

56 Schönfelder G, Wittfoht W, Hopp H, Talsness CE, Paul M, Chahoud I. Parent bisphenol A accumulation in the human maternal-fetal-placental unit. Environ Health Perspect. 2002 Nov;110(11):A703-7; Takahashi 2000; vom Saal 2007.

57 E.g. Cabaton, Nicolas J., Perinaaz R. Wadia, Beverly S. Rubin, Daniel Zalko, Cheryl M. Schaeberle, Michael H. Askenase, Jennifer L. Gadbois et al. "Perinatal exposure to environmentally relevant levels of bisphenol A decreases fertility and fecundity in CD-1 mice." Environmental health perspectives 119, no. 4 (2011): 547; Tharp, Andrew P., Maricel V. Maffini, Patricia A. Hunt, Catherine A. VandeVoort, Carlos Sonnenschein, and Ana M. Soto. "Bisphenol A alters the development of the rhesus monkey mammary gland." *Proceedings of the National Academy of Sciences* 109, no. 21 (2012): 8190-8195; Tian, Yu-Hua, Joung-Hee Baek, Seok-Yong Lee, and Choon-Gon Jang. "Prenatal and postnatal exposure to bisphenol a induces anxiolytic behaviors and cognitive deficits in mice." *Synapse* 64, no. 6 (2010): 432-439; Jang, Young Jung, Hee Ra Park, Tae Hyung Kim, Wook-Jin Yang, Jong-Joo Lee, Seon Young Choi, Shin Bi Oh et al. "High dose bisphenol A impairs hippocampal neurogenesis in female mice across generations." *Toxicology* (2012). Somm, Emmanuel, Valérie M. Schwitzgebel, Audrey Toulotte, Christopher R. Cederroth, Christophe Combescure, Serge Nef, Michel L. Aubert, and Petra S. Hüppi. "Perinatal exposure to bisphenol a alters early adipogenesis in the rat." *Environmental Health Perspectives* 117, no. 10 (2009): 1549. Braun, Joe M., Amy E. Kalkbrenner, Antonia M. Calafat, Kimberly Yolton, Xiaoyun Ye, Kim N. Dietrich, and Bruce P. Lanphear. "Impact of early-life bisphenol A exposure on behavior and executive function in children." *Pediatrics* 128, no. 5 (2011): 873-882.

58 Braun JM, Yolton K, Dietrich KN, Hornung R, Ye X, Calafat AM, Lanphear BP. Prenatal bisphenol A exposure and early childhood behavior. Environ Health Perspect. 2009 Dec;117(12):1945-52.

Chapter 3: Phthalates

1 Meeker JD, Sathyanarayana S, Swan SH.Phthalates and other additives in plastics: human exposure and associated health outcomes. Philos Trans R Soc Lond B Biol Sci. 2009 Jul 27;364(1526):2097-113.

2 Hauser R, Calafat AM. Phthalates and human health. Occup Environ Med. 2005 Nov;62(11):806-18.;

3 Directive 2005/84/EC of the European Parliament and of the Council of 14 December 2005.

4 U.S. Department of Health and Human Services, Food and Drug Administration, Center for Drug Evaluation and Research (CDER). Guidance for Industry: Limiting the Use of Certain Phthalates as Excipients in CDER-Regulated Products, December 2012.

5 David Byrne, EU Commissioner for Consumer Protection and Health, November 10th, 1999. http://europa.eu/rapid/press-release_IP-99-829_en.htm?locale=FR

6 Interview with EurActiv, 05/09/2012. http://www.euractiv.com/sustainability/us-scientist-routes-exposure-end-interview-512402

7 Berman T, Hochner-Celnikier D, Calafat AM, Needham LL, Amitai Y, Wormser U, et al. Phthalate exposure among pregnant women in Jerusalem, Israel: results of a pilot study. Environ Int. 2009;35:353-7.

8 Göen T, Dobler L, Koschorreck J, Müller J, Wiesmüller GA, Drexler H, Kolossa-Gehring M. Trends of the internal phthalate exposure of young adults in Germany—follow-up of a retrospective human biomonitoring study. Int J Hyg Environ Health. 2011 Dec;215(1):36-45.
Silva MJ, Barr DB, Reidy JA, Malek NA, Hodge CC, Caudill SP, Brock JW, Needham LL, Calafat AM. Urinary levels of seven phthalate metabolites in the U.S. population from the National Health and Nutrition Examination Survey (NHANES) 1999-2000. Environ Health Perspect. 2004 Mar;112(3):331-8.
Lin S, Ku HY, Su PH, Chen JW, Huang PC, Angerer J, Wang SL. Phthalate exposure in pregnant women and their children in central Taiwan. Chemosphere. 2011 Feb;82(7):947-55.

9 Davis BJ, Maronpot RR, Heindel JJ.Di-(2-ethylhexyl) phthalate suppresses estradiol and ovulation in cycling rats.Toxicol Appl Pharmacol. 1994 Oct;128(2):216-23.

10 Anas MK, Suzuki C, Yoshioka K, Iwamura S. Effect of mono-(2-ethylhexyl) phthalate on bovine oocyte maturation in vitro. Reprod Toxicol. 2003 May-Jun;17(3):305-10;
Ambruosi B, Uranio MF, Sardanelli AM, Pocar P, Martino NA, Paternoster MS, Amati F, Dell'Aquila ME. In vitro acute exposure to DEHP affects oocyte meiotic maturation, energy and oxidative stress parameters in a large animal model. PLoS One. 2011;6(11):e27452;
Grossman D, Kalo D, Gendelman M, Roth Z.Effect of di-(2-ethylhexyl) phthalate and mono-(2-ethylhexyl) phthalate on

in vitro developmental competence of bovine oocytes.Cell Biol Toxicol. 2012 Dec;28(6):383-96. ("Grossman 2012").

Gupta RK, Singh JM, Leslie TC, Meachum S, Flaws JA, Yao HH. Di-(2-ethylhexyl) phthalate and mono-(2-ethylhexyl) phthalate inhibit growth and reduce estradiol levels of antral follicles in vitro. Toxicol Appl Pharmacol. 2010 Jan 15;242(2):224-30. ("Gupta 2010").

11 Huang XF, Li Y, Gu YH, Liu M, Xu Y, Yuan Y, Sun F, Zhang HQ, Shi HJ. The effects of Di-(2-ethylhexyl)-phthalate exposure on fertilization and embryonic development in vitro and testicular genomic mutation in vivo. PLoS One. 2012;7(11):e50465.

Pant N, Pant A, Shukla M, Mathur N, Gupta Y, Saxena D. Environmental and experimental exposure of phthalate esters: the toxicological consequence on human sperm. Hum Exp Toxicol. 2011 Jun;30(6):507-14.

12 Duty S. M., Singh N. P., Silva M. J., Barr D. B., Brock J. W., Ryan L., Herrick R. F., Christiani D. C., Hauser R. 2003b. The relationship between environmental exposures to phthalates and DNA damage in human sperm using the neutral comet assay. Environ. Health Perspect. 111, 1164–1169. ("In conclusion, this study represents the first human data to demonstrate that urinary MEP, at environmental levels, is associated with increased DNA damage in sperm.")

13 Gupta 2010; Grossman 2012

14 Gupta 2010; Grossman 2012.

15 Reinsberg J, Wegener-Toper P, van der Ven K, van der Ven H, Klingmueller D. Effect of mono-(2-ethylhexyl) phthalate on steroid production of human granulosa cells. Toxicol Appl Pharmacol. 2009 Aug 15;239(1):116-23.

16 Lenie S, Smitz J. Steroidogenesis-disrupting compounds can be effectively studied for major fertility-related endpoints using in vitro cultured mouse follicles. Toxicol Lett. 2009 Mar 28;185(3):143-52.

17 Dalman A, Eimani H, Sepehri H, Ashtiani SK, Valojerdi MR, Eftekhari-Yazdi P, Shahverdi A. Effect of mono-(2-ethylhexyl) phthalate (MEHP) on resumption of meiosis, in vitro maturation and embryo development of immature mouse oocytes. Biofactors. 2008;33(2):149-55. ("Dalman 2008").

18 Grossman 2012.

19 Dalman 2008.

20 Hong YC, Park EY, Park MS, Ko JA, Oh SY, Kim H, Lee KH, Leem JH, Ha EH. Community level exposure to chemicals and oxidative stress in adult population. Toxicol. Lett. 2009;184(2):139–144;

Ferguson KK, Loch-Caruso R, Meeker JD.Urinary phthalate metabolites in relation to biomarkers of inflammation and oxidative stress: NHANES 1999-2006.Environ Res. 2011 Jul;111(5):718-26. ("Ferguson 2011").

21 Agarwal A, Gupta S, Sekhon L, Shah R. Redox considerations in female reproductive function and assisted reproduction: from molecular mechanisms to health implications. Antioxid Redox Signal. 2008 Aug;10(8):1375-403.

Zhang X, Wu XQ, Lu S, Guo YL, Ma X.Deficit of mitochondria-derived ATP during oxidative stress impairs mouse MII oocyte spindles.Cell Res. 2006 Oct;16(10):841-50.

22 Agarwal A, Aponte-Mellado A, Premkumar BJ, Shaman A, Gupta S. The effects of oxidative stress on female reproduction: a review. Reprod Biol Endocrinol. 2012 Jun 29;10:49

Ruder EH, Hartman TJ, Goldman MB. Impact of oxidative stress on female fertility. Curr Opin Obstet Gynecol. 2009 Jun;21(3):219-22.

Al-Gubory KH, Fowler PA, Garrel C. The roles of cellular reactive oxygen species, oxidative stress and antioxidants in pregnancy outcomes. Int J Biochem Cell Biol. 2010; 42:1634–1650.

23 Ferguson 2011.

24 Liu K, Lehmann KP, Sar M, Young SS, Gaido KW. Gene expression profiling following in utero exposure to phthalate esters reveals new gene targets in the etiology of testicular dysgenesis. Biol Reprod. 2005; 73:180–192.

Botelho GG, Bufalo AC, Boareto AC, Muller JC, Morais RN, Martino-Andrade AJ, Lemos KR, Dalsenter PR. Vitamin C and resveratrol supplementation to rat dams treated with di(2-ethylhexyl)phthalate: impact on reproductive and oxidative stress end points in male offspring. Arch Environ Contam Toxicol. 2009; 57:785–793

Erkekoglu P, Rachidi W, Yuzugullu OG, Giray B, Favier A, Ozturk M, Hincal F. Evaluation of cytotoxicity and oxidative DNA damaging effects of di(2-ethylhexyl)-phthalate (DEHP) and mono(2-ethylhexyl)-phthalate (MEHP) on MA-10 Leydig cells and protection by selenium. Toxicol Appl Pharmacol. 2010; 248:52–62.

25 Wang W, Craig ZR, Basavarajappa MS, Gupta RK, Flaws JA. Di (2-ethylhexyl) phthalate inhibits growth of mouse ovarian antral follicles through an oxidative stress pathway. Toxicol Appl Pharmacol. 2012 Jan 15;258(2):288-95. ("Wang 2012"); C.f. Ambruosi 2011.

26 Hauser R, Gaskins AJ, Souter I, Smith KW, Dodge LE, Ehrlich S, Meeker JD, Calafat AM, Williams PL, EARTH Study Team. Urinary phthalate metabolite concentrations and reproductive outcomes among women undergoing in vitro fertilization: results from the EARTH study. Environmental Health Perspectives. 2016 Jun 1;124(6):831.

27 Kim SH, Chun S, Jang JY, Chae HD, Kim CH, Kang BM. Increased plasma levels of phthalate esters in women with advanced-stage endometriosis: a prospective case-control study. Fertil Steril. 2011 Jan;95(1):357-9.
Reddy BS, Rozati R, Reddy S, Kodampur S, Reddy P, Reddy R. High plasma concentrations of polychlorinated biphenyls and phthalate esters in women with endometriosis: a prospective case control study. Fertil Steril. 2006 Mar;85(3):775-9;
Weuve J, Hauser R, Calafat AM, Missmer SA, Wise LA. Association of exposure to phthalates with endometriosis and uterine leiomyomata: findings from NHANES, 1999-2004. Environ Health Perspect. 2010 Jun;118(6):825-32.

28 Buck Louis GM, Peterson CM, Chen Z, Croughan M, Sundaram R, Stanford J, Varner MW, Kennedy A, Giudice L, Fujimoto VY, Sun L, Wang L, Guo Y, Kannan K.Bisphenol A and phthalates and endometriosis: the Endometriosis: Natural History, Diagnosis and Outcomes Study .Fertil Steril. 2013 Jul;100(1):162-9.e1-2.

29 Toft G, Jönsson BA, Lindh CH, Jensen TK, Hjollund NH, Vested A, Bonde JP. Association between pregnancy loss and urinary phthalate levels around the time of conception. Environ Health Perspect. 2012 Mar;120(3):458-63.

30 Latini G, et al. In utero exposure to di-(2-ethylhexyl)phthalate and duration of human pregnancy. Environmental Health Perspectives. 2003;111:1783–1785.
Meeker JD, Hu H, Cantonwine DE, Lamadrid-Figueroa H, Calafat AM, Ettinger AS, Hernandez-Avila M, Loch-Caruso R, Téllez-Rojo MM. Urinary phthalate metabolites in relation to preterm birth in Mexico city. Environ. Health Perspect. 2009;117(10):1587–1592.
Whyatt RM, Adibi JJ, Calafat AM, Camann DE, Rauh V, Bhat HK, Perera FP, Andrews H, Just AC, Hoepner L, Tang D, Hauser R. Prenatal di(2-ethylhexyl) phthalate exposure and length of gestation among an inner-city cohort. Pediatrics. 2009;124(6):e1213–e1220.

31 Meeker JD, Hu H, Cantonwine DE, Lamadrid-Figueroa H, Calafat AM, Ettinger AS, Hernandez-Avila M, Loch-Caruso R, Téllez-Rojo

MM. Urinary phthalate metabolites in relation to preterm birth in Mexico city. Environ. Health Perspect. 2009;117(10):1587–1592.

32 Latini G, Del Vecchio A, Massaro M, Verrotti A, De Felice C. In utero exposure to phthalates and fetal development. Curr Med Chem. 2006;13:2527–2534.

33 Meeker JD, Hu H, Cantonwine DE, Lamadrid-Figueroa H, Calafat AM, Ettinger AS, Hernandez-Avila M, Loch-Caruso R, Téllez-Rojo MM. Urinary phthalate metabolites in relation to preterm birth in Mexico city. Environ. Health Perspect. 2009;117(10):1587–1592.

34 Swan SH, Main KM, Liu F, Stewart SL, Kruse RL, Calafat AM, Mao CS, Redmon JB, Ternand CL, Sullivan S, Teague JL; Study for Future Families Research Team.Decrease in anogenital distance among male infants with prenatal phthalateexposure. Environ Health Perspect. 2005 Aug;113(8):1056-61. Erratum in: Environ Health Perspect. 2005 Sep;113(9):A583. ("Swan 2005").
Swan SH. Environmental phthalate exposure in relation to reproductive outcomes and other health endpoints in humans. Environ Res. 2008 Oct; 108(2):177-84.

35 Welsh M, et al. Identification in rats of a programming window for reproductive tract masculinization, disruption of which leads to hypospadias and cryptorchidism. The Journal of Clinical Investigation. 2008;118:1479–1490.
Foster P. M. 2006. Disruption of reproductive development in male rat offspring following *in utero* exposure to phthalate esters. Int. J. Androl. 29, 140–147 ("Foster 2006").

36 Swan 2005.

37 Interview with Dr. Shanna Swan, 06/12/2009, http://www.epa.gov/ nisujrgd/multimedia/audio/ehp_061209_transcript.html

38 Foster 2006.
Howdeshell KL, Wilson VS, Furr J, Lambright CR, Rider CV, Blystone CR, Hotchkiss AK, Gray LE Jr. A mixture of five phthalate esters inhibits fetal testicular testosterone production in the sprague-dawley rat in a cumulative, dose-additive manner. Toxicol Sci. 2008 Sep;105(1):153-65.

39 Akingbemi BT, Ge R, Klinefelter GR, Zirkin BR, Hardy MP. Phthalate-induced Leydig cell hyperplasia is associated with multiple endocrine disturbances. Proc Natl Acad Sci U S A. 2004 Jan 20;101(3):775-80;
Borch J, Ladefoged O, Hass U, Vinggaard AM. Steroidogenesis in fetal male rats is reduced by DEHP and DINP, but endocrine effects of DEHP are not modulated by DEHA in fetal, prepubertal and adult male rats. Reprod Toxicol. 2004 Jan-Feb;18(1):53-61;

Klinefelter GR, Laskey JW, Winnik WM, Suarez JD, Roberts NL, Strader LF, Riffle BW, Veeramachaneni DN. Novel molecular targets associated with testicular dysgenesis induced by gestational exposure to diethylhexyl phthalate in the rat: a role for estradiol. Reproduction. 2012 Dec; 144(6):747-61.

40 Whyatt RM, Liu X, Rauh VA, Calafat AM, Just AC, Hoepner L, Diaz D, Quinn J, Adibi J, Perera FP, Factor-Litvak P. Maternal prenatal urinary phthalate metabolite concentrations and child mental, psychomotor, and behavioral development at 3 years of age. Environ Health Perspect 2012;120:290 ("Whyatt 2012").

41 Yolton K, Xu Y, Strauss D, Altaye M, Calafat AM, Khoury J. Prenatal exposure to bisphenol A and phthalates and infant neurobehavior. Neurotoxicol Teratol 2011;33:558-66; Engel SM, Zhu C, Berkowitz GS, Calafat AM, Silva MJ, Miodovnik A, Wolff MS. Prenatal phthalate exposure and performance on the Neonatal Behavioral Assessment Scale in a multiethnic birth cohort. Neurotoxicology 2009;30:522-8; Kim Y, Ha EH, Kim EJ, Park H, Ha M, Kim JH, Hong YC, Chang N, Kim BN. Prenatal exposure to phthalates and infant development at 6 months: prospective Mothers and Children's Environmental Health (MOCEH) study. Environ Health Perspect 2011;119:1495-500; Engel SM, Miodovnik A, Canfield RL, Zhu C, Silva MJ, Calafat AM, Wolff MS. Prenatal phthalate exposure is associated with childhood behavior and executive functioning. Environ Health Perspect 2010;118:565-71; Swan SH, Liu F, Hines M, Kruse RL, Wang C, Redmon JB, Sparks A, Weiss B. Prenatal phthalate exposure and reduced masculine play in boys. Int J Androl 2010;33:259-69; Miodovnik A, Engel SM, Zhu C, Ye X, Soorya LV, Silva MJ, Calafat AM, Wolff MS. Endocrine disruptors and childhood social impairment. Neurotoxicology 2011;32:261-7; Whyatt 2012.

42 Boas M, Frederiksen H, Feldt-Rasmussen UF, Skakkebaek NE, Hegedus L, Hilsted, L, et al. Childhood exposure to phthalates: association with thyroid function, insulin-like growth factor I, and growth. Environ Health Perspect 2010; 118:1458–1464. Meeker and Ferguson 2011; Meeker JD, Ferguson KK. 2011. Relationship between urinary phthalate and bisphenol A concentrations and serum thyroid measures in U.S. adults and adolescents from the National Health and Nutrition Examination

Survey (NHANES) 2007–2008. Environ Health Perspect 119:1396–1402.

Meeker JD, Calafat AM, Hauser R. 2007. Di(2-ethylhexyl) phthalate metabolites may alter thyroid hormone levels in men. Environ Health Perspect 115:1029–1034.

43 Whyatt 2012.

44 Huang PC, Kuo PL, Guo YL, Liao PC, Lee CC. 2007. Associations between urinary phthalate monoesters and thyroid hormones in pregnant women. Hum Reprod 22(10):2715–2722.

45 Bornehag C. G., Sundell J., Weschler C. J., Sigsgaard T., Lundgren B., Hasselgren M., Hagerhed-Engman L. 2004. The association between asthma and allergic symptoms in children and phthalates in house dust: a nested case–control study. Environ. Health Perspect. 112, 1393–1397.
Kolarik B, et al. The association between phthalates in dust and allergic diseases among Bulgarian children. Environmental Health Perspectives. 2008;116:98–103.

46 Larsson M, Hägerhed-Engman L, Kolarik B, James P, Lundin F, Janson S, Sundell J, Bornehag CG. PVC—as flooring material— and its association with incident asthma in a Swedish child cohort study. Indoor Air. 2010 Dec;20(6):494-501.

47 Wormuth M, et al. What Are the Sources of Exposure to Eight Frequently Used Phthalic Acid Esters in Europeans? Risk Analysis. 2006;26:803–824. ("Wormuth 2006").

48 Sathyanarayana S., Karr C. J., Lozano P., Brown E., Calafat A. M., Liu F., Swan S. H. 2008. Baby care products: possible sources of infant phthalate exposure. Pediatrics 121, e260–e268

49 Koniecki D, Wang R, Moody RP, Zhu J.Phthalates in cosmetic and personal care products: concentrations and possible dermal exposure.Environ Res. 2011Apr;111(3):329-36. ("Koniecki 2011").
Janjua NR, Mortensen GK, Andersson AM, Kongshoj B, Skakkebaek NE, Wulf HC.Systemic uptake of diethyl phthalate, dibutyl phthalate, and butyl paraben following whole-body topical application and reproductive and thyroid hormone levels in humans. Environ Sci Technol. 2007 Aug 1;41(15):5564-70.

50 Wittassek M, Koch HM, Angerer J, Bruning T. Assessing exposure to phthalates – the human biomonitoring approach. Mol Nutr Food Res. 2011;55:7-31

51 Plenge-Bönig A, Karmaus W. Exposure to toluene in the printing industry is associated with subfecundity in women but not in men. Occup Environ Med. 1999 Jul;56(7):443-8.

Svensson BG, Nise G, Erfurth EM, Nilsson A, Skerfving S. Hormone status in occupational toluene exposure. Am J Ind Med. 1992;22(1):99–107.

Ng TP, Foo SC, Yoong T. Risk of spontaneous abortion in workers exposed to toluene. Br J Ind Med. 1992 Nov;49(11):804–808; Taskinen HK, Kyyrönen P, Sallmén M, Virtanen SV, Liukkonen TA, Huida O, Lindbohm ML, Anttila A. Reduced fertility among female wood workers exposed to formaldehyde. Am J Ind Med. 1999 Jul;36(1):206-12.

52 Lindbohm ML, Hemminki K, Bonhomme MG, Anttila A, Rantala K, Heikkila P, Rosenberg MJ. Effects of paternal occupational exposure on spontaneous abortions. American Journal of Public Health. 1991;81:1029–1033
Saurel-Cubizolles MJ, Hays M, Estryn-Behar M. Work in operating rooms and pregnancy outcome among nurses. Int Arch Occup Environ Health. 1994;66:235–241.
John EM, Savitz DA, Shy CM. Spontaneous abortions among cosmetologists. Epidemiology. 1994;5:147–155.

53 Koniecki 2011.

54 Wormuth 2006.

55 Koniecki 2011.

56 Wormuth 2006.

57 Colacino JA, Harris TR, Schecter A. Dietary intake is associated with phthalate body burden in a nationally representative sample. Environ Health Perspect. 2010 Jul;118(7):998-1003

58 Rudel RA, Gray JM, Engel CL, Rawsthorne TW, Dodson RE, Ackerman JM, Rizzo J, Nudelman JL, Brody JG. Food packaging and bisphenol A and bis(2-ethyhexyl) phthalate exposure: findings from a dietary intervention. Environ Health Perspect. 2011 Jul;119(7):914-20.

59 Montuori P, Jover E, Morgantini M, Bayona JM, Triassi M. Assessing human exposure to phthalic acid and phthalate esters from mineral water stored in polyethylene terephthalate and glass bottles. Food Add Contamin. 2008;25(4):511–518;
Sax L. Polyethylene terephthalate may yield endocrine disruptors. Environ Health Perspect. 2010;118:445–8;
Farhoodi M, Emam-Djomeh Z, Ehsani MR, Oromiehie A. Effect of environmental conditions on the migration of di(2-ethylhexyl) phthalate from PET bottles into yogurt drinks: influence of time, temperature, and food simulant. Arabian J Sci Eng. 2008;33(2):279–287.

60 Trasande L, Sathyanarayana S, Jo Messito M, S Gross R, Attina TM, Mendelsohn AL. Phthalates and the diets of US children and adolescents. Environ Res. 2013 Oct;126:84-90

61 Thornton, J, "Environmental impacts of polyvinyl chloride (PVC) building materials." briefing paper for the Healthy Building Network, http://www. healthybuilding. net/pvc/ ThorntonPVCSummary. html (2002).

62 Smith KW, Souter I, Dimitriadis I, Ehrlich S, Williams PL, Calafat AM, Hauser R. Urinary paraben concentrations and ovarian aging among women from a fertility center. Environ Health Perspect 2013 Aug;121:1299–1305.

63 http://www.ewg.org/research/dirty-dozen-list-endocrine-disruptors

64 http://www.ewg.org/report/ewgs-water-filter-buying-guide

65 Dr. Patricia Hunt, personal communication 02/06/2014.

66 Interview with EurActiv, 05/09/2012. http://www.euractiv.com/sustainability/us-scientist-routes-exposure-end-interview-512402

Chapter 4: Unexpected Obstacles to Fertility

1 Aleyasin A, Hosseini MA, Mahdavi A, Safdarian L, Fallahi P, Mohajeri MR, Abbasi M, Esfahani F.Predictive value of the level of vitamin D in follicular fluid on the outcome of assisted reproductive technology.Eur J Obstet Gynecol Reprod Biol. 2011 Nov;159(1):132-7.
Anifandis GM, Dafopoulos K, Messini CI, Chalvatzas N, Liakos N, Pournaras S, Messinis IE. Prognostic value of follicular fluid 25-OH vitamin D and glucose levels in the IVF outcome. Reprod Biol Endocrinol. 2010 Jul 28;8;91.

2 Rudick B, Ingles S, Chung K, Stanczyk F, Paulson R, Bendikson K. Characterizing the influence of vitamin D levels on IVF outcomes. Hum Reprod. 2012 Nov;27(11):3321-7. ("Rudick 2012").

3 Ozkan S, Jindal S, Greenseid K, Shu J, Zeitlian G, Hickmon C, Pal L. Replete vitamin D stores predict reproductive success following in vitro fertilization. Fertil Steril. 2010 Sep;94(4):1314-9.

4 Firouzabadi RD, Rahmani E, Rahsepar M, Firouzabadi MM. Value of follicular fluid vitamin D in predicting the pregnancy rate in an IVF program. Arch Gynecol Obstet. 2014 Jan;289(1):201-6

5 Ruddick 2012). Rudick B, Ingles S, Chung K, Stanczyk F, Paulson R, Bendikson K. Characterizing the influence of vitamin D levels on IVF outcomes. Hum Reprod. 2012 Nov;27(11):3321-7.

6 Luk J, Torrealday S, Neal Perry G, Pal L. Relevance of vitamin D in reproduction. Hum Reprod. 2012 Oct;27(10):3015-27 ("Luk 2012").

7 Luk 2012.

8 Looker AC, Pfeiffer CM, Lacher DA, Schleicher RL, Picciano MF, Yetley EA. Serum 25-hydroxyvitamin D status of the US population: 1988-1994 compared with 2000-2004. Am J Clin Nutr. 2008 Dec;88(6):1519-27 ("Looker 2008"); Nesby-O'Dell S, Scanlon KS, Cogswell ME, Gillespie C, Hollis BW, Looker AC, Allen C, Doughertly C, Gunter EW, Bowman BA. Hypovitaminosis D prevalence and determinants among African American and white women of reproductive age: third National Health and Nutrition Examination Survey, 1988-1994. Am J Clin Nutr. 2002 Jul;76(1):187-92

9 Looker 2008

10 Luk 2012

11 Grundmann M, von Versen-Höynck F. Vitamin D - roles in women's reproductive health? Reprod Biol Endocrinol. 2011 Nov 2;9:146.

12 Li HW, Brereton RE, Anderson RA, Wallace AM, Ho CK. Vitamin D deficiency is common and associated with metabolic risk factors in patients with polycystic ovary syndrome. Metabolism. 2011 Oct;60(10):1475-81

13 Wehr E, Pilz S, Schweighofer N, Giuliani A, Kopera D, Pieber TR, Obermayer-Pietsch B. Association of hypovitaminosis D with metabolic disturbances in polycystic ovary syndrome. Eur J Endocrinol. 2009 Oct;161(4):575-82.

14 Wehr E, Pieber TR, Obermayer-Pietsch B. Effect of vitamin D3 treatment on glucose metabolism and menstrual frequency in polycystic ovary syndrome women: a pilot study. J Endocrinol Invest. 2011 Nov;34(10):757-63.

15 Grossmann RE, Tangpricha V. Evaluation of vehicle substances on vitamin D bioavailability: a systematic review. Mol Nutr Food Res. 2010 Aug;54(8):1055-61;
Raimundo FV, Faulhaber GA, Menegatti PK, Marques Lda S, Furlanetto TW. Effect of High- versus Low-Fat Meal on Serum 25-Hydroxyvitamin D Levels after a Single Oral Dose of Vitamin D: A Single-Blind, Parallel, Randomized Trial. Int J Endocrinol. 2011;2011:809069.

16 Stagnaro-Green A, Roman SH, Cobin RH, el-Harazy E, Alvarez-Marfany M, Davies TF. Detection of at-risk pregnancy by means of highly sensitive assays for thyroid autoantibodies. JAMA. 1990 Sep 19;264(11):1422-5 ("Stagnaro-Green 1990");
Thangaratinam S, Tan A, Knox E, Kilby MD, Franklyn J, Coomarasamy A. Association between thyroid autoantibodies and

miscarriage and preterm birth: meta-analysis of evidence. BMJ. 2011 May 9;342:d2616. ("Thangaratinam 2011").

17 Stagnaro-Green 1990.

18 Stagnaro-Green A. Thyroid antibodies and miscarriage: where are we at a generation later? J Thyroid Res. 2011; 2011:841949.

19 Ghafoor F, Mansoor M, Malik T, Malik MS, Khan AU, Edwards R, Akhtar W. Role of thyroid peroxidase antibodies in the outcome of pregnancy. J Coll Physicians Surg Pak. 2006 Jul;16(7):468-71.

20 Pratt DE, Kaberlein G, Dudkiewicz A, Karande V, Gleicher N. The association of antithyroid antibodies in euthyroid nonpregnant women with recurrent first trimester abortions in the next pregnancy. Fertil Steril. 1993 Dec;60(6):1001-5;
Bussen S, Steck T. Thyroid autoantibodies in euthyroid non-pregnant women with recurrent spontaneous abortions. Hum Reprod. 1995 Nov;10(11):2938-40;
Dendrinos S, Papasteriades C, Tarassi K, Christodoulakos G, Prasinos G, Creatsas G. Thyroid autoimmunity in patients with recurrent spontaneous miscarriages. Gynecol Endocrinol. 2000 Aug;14(4):270-4.

21 Toulis KA, Goulis DG, Venetis CA, Kolibianakis EM, Negro R, Tarlatzis BC, Papadimas I. Risk of spontaneous miscarriage in euthyroid women with thyroid autoimmunity undergoing IVF: a meta-analysis. Eur J Endocrinol. 2010 Apr;162(4):643-52;
Prummel MF, Wiersinga WM. Thyroid autoimmunity and miscarriage. Eur J Endocrinol. 2004 Jun;150(6):751-5;
Thangaratinam 2011

22 Negro R, Schwartz A, Gismondi R, Tinelli A, Mangieri T, Stagnaro-Green A. Increased pregnancy loss rate in thyroid antibody negative women with TSH levels between 2.5 and 5.0 in the first trimester of pregnancy. J Clin Endocrinol Metab. 2010 Sep;95(9):E44-8. ("Negro 2010").

23 Negro 2010.

24 Negro R, Formoso G, Mangieri T, Pezzarossa A, Dazzi D, Hassan H. Levothyroxine treatment in euthyroid pregnant women with autoimmune thyroid disease: effects on obstetrical complications. J Clin Endocrinol Metab. 2006 Jul;91(7):2587-91.

25 Kim CH, Ahn JW, Kang SP, Kim SH, Chae HD, Kang BM. Effect of levothyroxine treatment on in vitro fertilization and pregnancy outcome in infertile women with subclinical hypothyroidism undergoing in vitro fertilization/intracytoplasmic sperm injection. Fertil Steril. 2011 Apr;95(5):1650-4. ("Kim 2011").

26 Abalovich M, Mitelberg L, Allami C, Gutierrez S, Alcaraz G, Otero P, Levalle O. Subclinical hypothyroidism and thyroid autoimmunity in women with infertility. Gynecol Endocrinol. 2007 May;23(5):279-83. ("Abalovich 2007").

27 Eldar-Geva T, Shoham M, Rösler A, Margalioth EJ, Livne K, Meirow D. Subclinical hypothyroidism in infertile women: the importance of continuous monitoring and the role of the thyrotropin-releasing hormone stimulation test. Gynecol Endocrinol. 2007 Jun;23(6):332-7.

28 Abalovich 2007

29 Kim 2011.

30 Janssen OE, Mehlmauer N, Hahn S, Offner AH, Gärtner R. High prevalence of autoimmune thyroiditis in patients with polycystic ovary syndrome. Eur J Endocrinol. 2004 Mar;150(3):363-9. Sinha U, Sinharay K, Saha S, Longkumer TA, Baul SN, Pal SK. Thyroid disorders in polycystic ovarian syndrome subjects: A tertiary hospital based cross-sectional study from Eastern India .Indian J Endocrinol Metab. 2013 Mar;17(2):304-9.

31 Fasano A, Catassi C. Current Approaches to Diagnosis and Treatment of Celiac Disease: An Evolving Spectrum. Gastroenterology, 2001;120:636-651.

32 Kaukinen K, Maki M, Collin P. Immunohistochemical features in antiendomysium positive patients with normal villous architecture. Am J Gastroenterol, 2006;101(3):675-676; Kumar V. American Celiac Society, Nov.9,1999.

33 Pellicano R., Astegiano M., Bruno M., Fagoonee S., Rizzetto M.. Women and celiac disease: association with unexplained infertility. Minerva Med, 2007;98:217-219. ("Pellicano 2007").

34 Ferguson R, Holmes GK, Cooke WT. Coeliac disease, fertility, and pregnancy. Scand J Gastroenterol, 1982;17:65–68.

35 Choi JM, Lebwohl B, Wang J, Lee SK, Murray JA, Sauer MV, Green PH. Increased prevalence of celiac disease in patients with unexplained infertility in the United States.J Reprod Med. 2011 May-Jun;56(5-6):199-203. ("Choi 2011"); Kumar A, Meena M, Begum N, Kumar N, Gupta RK, Aggarwal S, Prasad S, Batra S. Latent celiac disease in reproductive performance of women. Fertil Steril. 2011 Mar 1;95(3):922-7; Machado AP, Silva LR, Zausner B, Oliveira Jde A, Diniz DR, de Oliveira J. Undiagnosed celiac disease in women with infertility. J Reprod Med. 2013 Jan-Feb;58(1-2):61-6; Pellicano 2007.

36 Jackson JE, Rosen M, McLean T, et al. Prevalence of celiac disease in a cohort of women with unexplained infertility. Fertil Steril. 2008; 89:1002–1004.
37 Choi 2011.
38 Ciacci C, Cirillo M, Auriemma G, Di Dato G, Sabbatini F, Mazzacca G. Celiac disease and pregnancy outcome. Am J Gastroenterol, 1996;91(4):718-722.
39 La Villa G, Pantaleo P, Tarquini R, Cirami L, Perfetto F, Mancuso F, Laffi G. Multiple immune disorders in unrecognized celiac disease: a case report. World J Gastroenterol, 2003;9(6): 1377-1380. ("La Villa 2003").
40 La Villa 2003.
41 Bast A, O'Bryan T, Bast E. Celiac Disease and Reproductive Health. Pract Gastroenterol. 2009 Oct:10-21 ("Bast 2009").
42 Pellicano 2007.
43 Dickey W, Ward M, Whittle CR, Kelly MT, Pentieva K, Horigan G, Patton S, McNulty H. Homocysteine and related B-vitamin status in coeliac disease: Effects of gluten exclusion and histological recovery. Scand J Gastroenterol. 2008;43(6):682-8. ("Dickey 2008").
44 Ocal 2012. Ocal P, Ersoylu B, Cepni I, Guralp O, Atakul N, Irez T, Idil M.The association between homocysteine in the follicular fluid with embryo quality and pregnancy rate in assisted reproductive techniques. J Assist Reprod Genet. 2012 Apr;29(4):299-304.
45 Dickey 2008.
46 Hallert C, Grant C, Grehn S, Grännö C, Hultén S, Midhagen G, Ström M, Svensson H, Valdimarsson T.Evidence of poor vitamin status in coeliac patients on a gluten-free diet for 10 years. Aliment Pharmacol Ther. 2002 Jul;16(7):1333-9.
47 Hallert C, Svensson M, Tholstrup J, Hultberg B.Clinical trial: B vitamins improve health in patients with coeliac disease living on a gluten-free diet. Aliment Pharmacol Ther. 2009 Apr 15;29(8):811-6.
48 Choi 2011.
49 Bast 2009.
50 Ide M, Papapanou PN. Epidemiology of association between maternal periodontal disease and adverse pregnancy outcomes—systematic review. J Periodontol. 2013 Apr;84(4 Suppl):S181-94.
Vogt M, Sallum AW, Cecatti JG, Morais SS. Periodontal disease and some adverse perinatal outcomes in a cohort of low risk pregnant women. Reprod Health. 2010 Nov 3;7:29
Offenbacher S, Beck JD. Periodontitis: a potential risk factor for spontaneous preterm birth. Compend. Contin. Educ. Dent.22(2 Spec No),17–20 (2001).

Shub A, Wong C, Jennings B, Swain JR, Newnham JP. Maternal periodontal disease and perinatal mortality. Aust N Z J Obstet Gynaecol 2009;49:130-136.

51 Jeffcoat MK, Geurs NC, Reddy MS, Cliver SP, Goldenberg RL, Hauth JC. Periodontal infection and preterm birth: results of a prospective study. J Am Dent Assoc. 2001 Jul;132(7):875-80

52 Farrell S, Ide M, Wilson RF. The relationship between maternal periodontitis, adverse pregnancy outcome and miscarriage in never smokers. J Clin Periodontol. 2006 Feb;33(2):115-20.

53 Madianos PN, Bobetsis YA, Offenbacher S.Adverse pregnancy outcomes (APOs) and periodontal disease: pathogenic mechanisms.J Periodontol. 2013 Apr;84 (4 Suppl):S170-80.

54 Hart R, Doherty DA, Pennell CE, Newnham IA, Newnham JP. Periodontal disease: a potential modifiable risk factor limiting conception. Hum Reprod. 2012 May;27(5):1332-42.

55 Newnham JP, Newnham IA, Ball CM, Wright M, Pennell CE, Swain J, Doherty DA. Treatment of periodontal disease during pregnancy: a randomized controlled trial. Obstet Gynecol 2009;114:1239-1248.

Chapter 5: Prenatal Multivitamins

1 CDC, ten great public health achievements- United States, 2001-2010. Morb Mortal Wkly Rep 2011: 60-619-23.

2 Prevention of neural tube defects: results of the Medical Research Council Vitamin Study MRC Vitamin Study Research Group. Lancet. 1991 Jul 20;338(8760):131-7.

3 Smithells RW, Sheppard S, Schorah CJ, Seller MJ, Nevin NC, Harris R, Read AP, Fielding DW.Apparent prevention of neural tube defects by periconceptional vitamin supplementation. 1981.Int J Epidemiol. 2011 Oct;40(5):1146-54.

4 Schorah C. Commentary: from controversy and procrastination to primary prevention. Int J Epidemiol. 2011 Oct;40(5):1156-8. ("Schorah 2011").

5 Schorah 2011.

6 Czeizel AE, Dudás I. Prevention of the first occurrence of neural-tube defects by periconceptional vitamin supplementation. N Engl J Med. 1992 Dec 24;327(26):1832-5;
de Bree A, van Dusseldorp M, Brouwer IA, van het Hof KH, Steegers-Theunissen RP. Folate intake in Europe: recommended, actual and desired intake. Eur J Clin Nutr. 1997 Oct;51(10):643-60.

7 http://www.cdc.gov/ncbddd/folicacid/recommendations.html

http://www.nhs.uk/Conditions/vitamins-minerals/Pages/
Vitamin-B.aspx

8 http://www.uspreventiveservicestaskforce.org/uspstf09/folicacid/
folicacidrs.htm

9 Ebisch IM, Thomas CM, Peters WH, Braat DD, Steegers-
Theunissen RP. The importance of folate, zinc and antioxidants
in the pathogenesis and prevention of subfertility. Hum Reprod
Update. 2007 Mar-Apr;13(2):163-74 ("Ebisch 2007").

10 Chavarro JE, Rich-Edwards JW, Rosner BA, Willett WC. Use
of multivitamins, intake of B vitamins, and risk of ovulatory
infertility. Fertil Steril. 2008 Mar;89(3):668-76.

11 Westphal LM, Polan ML, Trant AS, Mooney SB. A nutritional
supplement for improving fertility in women: a pilot study. J
Reprod Med. 2004 Apr;49(4):289-93.
Czeizel AE, Métneki J, Dudás I. The effect of preconceptional
multivitamin supplementation on fertility. Int J Vitam Nutr Res.
1996;66(1):55-8.

12 Gaskins AJ, Mumford SL, Chavarro JE, Zhang C, Pollack AZ,
Wactawski-Wende J, Perkins NJ, Schisterman EF. The impact of
dietary folate intake on reproductive function in premenopausal
women: a prospective cohort study. PLoS One. 2012;7(9):e46276.
("Gaskins 2012").

13 Gaskins 2012.

14 Dudás I, Rockenbauer M, Czeizel AE. The effect of preconceptional
multivitamin supplementation on the menstrual cycle. Arch
Gynecol Obstet. 1995;256(3):115-23.

15 Ebisch 2007.

16 Boxmeer JC, Brouns RM, Lindemans J, Steegers EA, Martini E,
Macklon NS, Steegers-Theunissen RP. Preconception folic acid
treatment affects the microenvironment of the maturing oocyte in
humans. Fertil Steril. 2008 Jun;89(6):1766-70. ("Boxmeer 2008").

17 Enciso M, Sarasa J, Xanthopoulou L, Bristow S, Bowles M, Fragouli
E, Delhanty J, Wells D. Polymorphisms in the MTHFR gene
influence embryo viability and the incidence of aneuploidy. Human
genetics. 2016 May 1;135(5):555-68.

18 Hekmatdoost A, Vahid F, Yari Z, Sadeghi M, Eini-Zinab H,
Lakpour N, Arefi S. Methyltetrahydrofolate vs Folic Acid
Supplementation in Idiopathic Recurrent Miscarriage with Respect
to Methylenetetrahydrofolate Reductase C677T and A1298C
Polymorphisms: A Randomized Controlled Trial. PloS one. 2015
Dec 2;10(12):e0143569.

19 National Institutes of Health Dietary Supplement Fact Sheet, Folate https://ods.od.nih.gov/factsheets/Folate-HealthProfessional/#en2

20 Boxmeer JC, Macklon NS, Lindemans J, Beckers NG, Eijkemans MJ, Laven JS, Steegers EA, Steegers-Theunissen RP. IVF outcomes are associated with biomarkers of the homocysteine pathway in monofollicular fluid. Hum Reprod. 2009 May;24(5):1059-66.

Chapter 6: The Power of Coenzyme Q10

1 Dietmar A, Schmidt ME, Siebrecht SC. Ubiquinol supplementation enhances peak power production in trained athletes: a double-blind, placebo controlled study. J Int Soc Sports Nutr. 2013 Apr 29;10(1):24.

2 Bentinger M, Brismar K, Dallner G. The antioxidant role of coenzyme Q. Mitochondrion. 2007 Jun;7 Suppl:S41-50;
Sohal RS. Coenzyme Q and vitamin E interactions. Methods Enzymol. 2004;378:146-51.

3 Shigenaga MK, Hagen TM, Ames BN.Oxidative damage and mitochondrial decay in aging.Proc Natl Acad Sci U S A. 1994 Nov 8;91(23):10771-8.
Seo AY, Joseph AM, Dutta D, Hwang JC, Aris JP, Leeuwenburgh C.New insights into the role of mitochondria in aging: mitochondrial dynamics and more.J Cell Sci. 2010 Aug 1;123(Pt 15):2533-42 ("Seo 2010").

4 Seo 2010

5 Tatone C, Amicarelli F, Carbone MC, Monteleone P, Caserta D, Marci R, Artini PG, Piomboni P, Focarelli R. Cellular and molecular aspects of ovarian follicle ageing. Hum Reprod Update. 2008 Mar-Apr;14(2):131-42.

6 Wilding M, Dale B, Marino M, di Matteo L, Alviggi C, Pisaturo ML, Lombardi L, De Placido G. Mitochondrial aggregation patterns and activity in human oocytes and preimplantation embryos. Hum Reprod. 2001 May;16(5):909-17 ("Wilding 2001").

7 de Bruin JP, Dorland M, Spek ER, Posthuma G, van Haaften M, Looman CW, te Velde ER. Age-related changes in the ultrastructure of the resting follicle pool in human ovaries. Biol Reprod. 2004 Feb;70(2):419-24 ("deBruin 2004").

8 Wilding 2001.

9 Bentov Y, Casper RF.The aging oocyte—can mitochondrial function be improved? Fertil Steril. 2013 Jan;99(1):18-22. ("Bentov 2013").

10 Bonomi M, Somigliana E, Cacciatore C, Busnelli M, Rossetti R, Bonetti S, Paffoni A, Mari D, Ragni G, Persani L; Italian Network

for the study of Ovarian Dysfunctions. Blood cell mitochondrial DNA content and premature ovarian aging. PLoS One. 2012;7(8):e42423

11 Van Blerkom J, Davis PW, Lee J. ATP content of human oocytes and developmental potential and outcome after in-vitro fertilization and embryo transfer. Hum Reprod. 1995 Feb;10(2):415-24

12 Santos TA, El Shourbagy A, St John JC. Mitochondrial content reflects oocyte variability and fertilization outcome. Fertil Steril. 2006;85:584–91;
Bentov Y, Esfandiari N, Burstein E, Casper RF.The use of mitochondrial nutrients to improve the outcome of infertility treatment in older patients.Fertil Steril.
2010 Jan;93(1):272-5 ("Bentov 2010").

13 Harvey AJ, Gibson TC, Quebedeaux TM, Brenner CA. Impact of assisted reproductive technologies: a mitochondrial perspective of cytoplasmic transplantation. Curr Top Dev Biol. 2007;77:229–49.

14 Dumollard R, Carroll J, Duchen MR, Campbell K, Swann K. Mitochondrial function and redox state in mammalian embryos. Semin Cell Dev Biol. 2009 May;20(3):346-53.

15 Van Blerkom J. Mitochondrial function in the human oocyte and embryo and their role in developmental competence. Mitochondrion. 2011 Sep;11(5):797-813 ("Van Blerkom 2011").

16 Eichenlaub-Ritter U, Vogt E, Yin H, Gosden R. Spindles, mitochondria and redox
potential in ageing oocytes. Reprod Biomed Online. 2004 Jan;8(1):45-58; Van Blerkom 2011;

17 Ge H, Tollner TL, Hu Z, Dai M, Li X, Guan H, Shan D, Zhang X, Lv J, Huang C, Dong Q. The importance of mitochondrial metabolic activity and mitochondrial DNA replication during oocyte maturation in vitro on oocyte quality and subsequent embryo developmental competence. Mol Reprod Dev. 2012 Jun;79(6):392-401.

18 Wilding M, Placido G, Matteo L, Marino M, Alviggi C, Dale B. Chaotic mosaicism in human preimplantation embryos is correlated with a low mitochondrial membrane potential. Fertil Steril. 2003;79:340–6 ("Wilding 2003").
Zeng HT, Ren Z, Yeung WS, Shu YM, Xu YW, Zhuang GL, Liang XY. Low mitochondrial DNA and ATP contents contribute to the absence of birefringent spindle imaged with PolScope in in vitro matured human oocytes. Hum Reprod. 2007 Jun;22(6):1681-6.

19 Yu Y, Dumollard R, Rossbach A, Lai FA, Swann K. Redistribution of mitochondria leads to bursts of ATP production during spontaneous mouse oocyte maturation. J Cell Physiol. 2010 Sep;224(3):672-80.

20 Wilding 2003.

21 Zhang X, Wu XQ, Lu S, Guo YL, Ma X. Deficit of mitochondria-derived ATP during oxidative stress impairs mouse MII oocyte spindles. Cell Res. 2006 Oct;16(10):841-50.

22 Eichenlaub-Ritter U, Vogt E, Yin H, Gosden R. Spindles, mitochondria and redox potential in ageing oocytes. Reprod Biomed Online. 2004 Jan;8(1):45-58.

23 Bartmann AK, Romao GS, Ramos Eda S, Ferriani RA. Why do older women have poor implantation rates? A possible role of the mitochondria. J Assist Reprod Genet. 2004;21:79-83; Thundathil J, Filion F, Smith LC.Molecular control of mitochondrial function in preimplantation mouse embryos.Mol Reprod Dev. 2005 Aug;71(4):405-13.

24 Thouas GA, Trounson AO, Wolvetang EJ, Jones GM. Mitochondrial dysfunction in mouse oocytes results in preimplantation embryo arrest in vitro. Biol Reprod. 2004 Dec;71(6):1936-42; Eichenlaub-Ritter U, Wieczorek M, Lüke S, Seidel T. Age related changes in mitochondrial function and new approaches to study redox regulation in mammalian oocytes in response to age or maturation conditions. Mitochondrion. 2011 Sep;11(5):783-96.

25 Interview with Dr. Bentov, published May 16, 2011, http://www.chatelaine.com/health/what-every-woman-over-30-should-know-about-fertility/

26 Bentov 2010; Bentov 2013.

27 Quinzii CM, Hirano M, DiMauro S. CoQ10 deficiency diseases in adults. Mitochondrion. 2007;7(Suppl):S122-6; Lopez 2010, Bergamini 2012, Shigenaga MK, Hagen TM, Ames BN. Oxidative damage and mitochondrial decay in aging. Proc Natl Acad Sci U S A. 1994 Nov 8;91(23):10771-8.

28 Perez-Sanchez C, Ruiz-Limon P, Aguirre MA, Bertolaccini ML, Khamashta MA, Rodriguez-Ariza A, Segui P, Collantes-Estevez E, Barbarroja N, Khraiwesh H, Gonzalez-Reyes JA, Villalba JM, Velasco F, Cuadrado MJ, Lopez-Pedrera C. Mitochondrial dysfunction in antiphospholipid syndrome: implications in the pathogenesis of the disease and effects of coenzyme Q(10) treatment. Blood. 2012 Jun 14;119(24):5859-70.

29 Stojkovic M, Westesen K, Zakhartchenko V, Stojkovic P, Boxhammer K, Wolf E.Coenzyme Q(10) in submicron-sized dispersion improves development, hatching, cell proliferation, and adenosine triphosphate content of in vitro-produced bovine embryos.biol Reprod. 1999 Aug;61(2):541-7.

30 Bentov 2013.

31 Bentov 2013.

32 Turi A, Giannubilo SR, Brugè F, Principi F, Battistoni S, Santoni F, Tranquilli AL, Littarru G, Tiano L.Coenzyme Q10 content in follicular fluid and its relationship with oocyte fertilization and embryo grading.Arch Gynecol Obstet. 2012 Apr;285(4):1173-6.

33 Bentov Y, Esfandiari N, Burstein E, Casper RF.The use of mitochondrial nutrients to improve the outcome of infertility treatment in older patients.Fertil Steril. 2010 Jan;93(1):272-5.

34 Kamei M, Fujita T, Kanbe T, Sasaki K, Oshiba K, Otani S, Matsui-Yuasa I, Morisawa S. The distribution and content of ubiquinone in foods. Int J Vitam Nutr Res. 1986;56(1):57-63.

35 Bhagavan HN, Chopra RK. Coenzyme Q10: absorption, tissue uptake, metabolism and pharmacokinetics. Free Radic Res. 2006 May;40(5):445-53 ("Bhagavan 2006").

36 Aberg F, Appelkvist EL, Dallner G, Ernster L. Distribution and redox state of ubiquinones in rat and human tissues. Arch Biochem Biophys. 1992 Jun;295(2):230-4;
Miles MV, Horn PS, Morrison JA, Tang PH, DeGrauw T, Pesce AJ. Plasma coenzyme Q10 reference intervals, but not redox status, are affected by gender and race in self-reported healthy adults. Clin Chim Acta. 2003 Jun;332(1-2):123-32.

37 Hosoe K, Kitano M, Kishida H, Kubo H, Fujii K, Kitahara M. Study on safety and bioavailability of ubiquinol (Kaneka QH) after single and 4-week multiple oral administration to healthy volunteers. Regul Toxicol Pharmacol. 2007 Feb;47(1):19-28 ("Hosoe 2007");
Ikematsu H, Nakamura K, Harashima S, Fujii K, Fukutomi N. Safety assessment of coenzyme Q10 (Kaneka Q10) in healthy subjects: a double-blind, randomized, placebo-controlled trial. Regul Toxicol Pharmacol. 2006 Apr;44(3):212-8.

38 Villalba JM, Parrado C, Santos-Gonzalez M, Alcain FJ. Therapeutic use of coenzyme Q10 and coenzyme Q10-related compounds and formulations. Expert Opin Investig Drugs. 2010 Apr;19(4):535-54.

39 Bergamini C, Moruzzi N, Sblendido A, Lenaz G, Fato R. A water soluble CoQ10 formulation improves intracellular distribution and promotes mitochondrial respiration in cultured cells. PLoS One.

2012;7(3):e33712; Chopra RK, Goldman R, Sinatra ST, Bhagavan HN. Relative bioavailability of coenzyme Q10 formulations in human subjects. Int J Vitam Nutr Res. 1998;68(2):109-13., Bhagavan 2006;

40 Spindler M, Beal MF, Henchcliffe C. Coenzyme Q10 effects in neurodegenerative disease. Neuropsychiatr Dis Treat. 2009;5:597-610 ("Spindler 2009"); Hosoe 2007.

41 Ferrante KL, Shefner J, Zhang H, Betensky R, O'Brien M, Yu H, Fantasia M, Taft J, Beal MF, Traynor B, Newhall K, Donofrio P, Caress J, Ashburn C, Freiberg B, O'Neill C, Paladenech C, Walker T, Pestronk A, Abrams B, Florence J, Renna R, Schierbecker J, Malkus B, Cudkowicz M. Tolerance of high-dose (3,000 mg/day) coenzyme Q10 in ALS. Neurology. 2005 Dec 13;65(11):1834-6; Spindler 2009.

42 Hosoe 2007.

43 Mezawa M, Takemoto M, Onishi S, Ishibashi R, Ishikawa T, Yamaga M, Fujimoto M, Okabe E, He P, Kobayashi K, Yokote K. The reduced form of coenzyme Q10 improves glycemic control in patients with type 2 diabetes: an open label pilot study. Biofactors. 2012 Nov-Dec;38(6):416-21.

44 Molyneux SL, Young JM, Florkowski CM, Lever M, George PM. Coenzyme Q10: is there a clinical role and a case for measurement? Clin Biochem Rev. 2008 May;29(2):71-82.

45 Hsoe 2007.

Chapter 7: Melatonin and Other Antioxidants

1 Evans H. The pioneer history of vitamin E. Vitam Horm. 1963;20:379–387.

2 de Bruin JP, Dorland M, Spek ER, Posthuma G, van Haaften M, Looman CW, te Velde ER. Age-related changes in the ultrastructure of the resting follicle pool in human ovaries. Biol Reprod. 2004 Feb;70(2):419-24. ("de Bruin 2004").

3 Tatone C, Carbone MC, Falone S, Aimola P, Giardinelli A, Caserta D, Marci R, Pandolfi A, Ragnelli AM, Amicarelli F. Age-dependent changes in the expression of superoxide dismutases and catalase are associated with ultrastructural modifications in human granulosa cells. Mol Hum Reprod. 2006 Nov;12(11):655-60. Carbone MC, Tatone C, Delle Monache S, Marci R, Caserta D, Colonna R, Amicarelli F. Antioxidant enzymatic defences in human follicular fluid: characterization and age-dependent changes. Mol Hum Reprod. 2003 Nov;9(11):639-43.

4 Shigenaga MK, Hagen TM, Ames BN.Oxidative damage and mitochondrial decay in aging. Proc Natl Acad Sci U S A. 1994 Nov 8;91(23):10771-8.

5 Agarwal A, Aponte-Mellado A, Premkumar BJ, Shaman A, Gupta S. The effects of oxidative stress on female reproduction: a review. Reprod Biol Endocrinol. 2012 Jun 29;10:49. ("Agarwal 2012.")

6 Bentov Y, Casper RF.The aging oocyte—can mitochondrial function be improved? Fertil Steril. 2013 Jan;99(1):18-22. ("Bentov 2013").

7 Polak G, Koziol-Montewka M, Gogacz M, Blaszkowska I, Kotarski J. Total antioxidant status of peritoneal fluid in infertile women. Eur J Obstet Gynecol Reprod Biol. 2001;94:261-263.
Wang Y, Sharma RK, Falcone T, Goldberg J, Agarwal A. Importance of reactive oxygen species in the peritoneal fluid of women with endometriosis or idiopathic infertility. Fertil Steril. 1997;68:826-830. ("Wang 1997").
Paszkowski T, Traub AI, Robinson SY, McMaster D. Selenium dependent glutathione peroxidase activity in human follicular fluid. Clin Chim Acta. 1995;236(2):173-180. doi: 10.1016/0009-8981(95)98130-9. ("Paszkowski 1995").

8 Kumar K, Deka D, Singh A, Mitra DK, Vanitha BR, Dada R.Predictive value of DNA integrity analysis in idiopathic recurrent pregnancy loss following spontaneous conception. J Assist Reprod Genet. 2012 Sep;29(9):861-7.

9 Zhang X, Wu XQ, Lu S, Guo YL, Ma X.Deficit of mitochondria-derived ATP during oxidative stress impairs mouse MII oocyte spindles.Cell Res. 2006 Oct;16(10):841-50.

10 Agarwal 2012; Wang 1997.

11 Augoulea A, Mastorakos G, Lambrinoudaki I, Christodoulakos G, Creatsas G. The role of the oxidative-stress in the endometriosis-related infertility. Gynecol Endocrinol. 2009;25:75-81.); Bedaiwy MA, Falcone T. Peritoneal fluid environment in endometriosis. clinicopathological implications. Minerva Ginecol. 2003;55:333-45.
Rajani S, Chattopadhyay R, Goswami SK, Ghosh S, Sharma S, Chakravarty B. Assessment of oocyte quality in polycystic ovarian syndrome and endometriosis by spindle imaging and reactive oxygen species levels in follicular fluid and its relationship with IVF-ET outcome. J Hum Reprod Sci. 2012 May;5(2):187-93. ("Rajani 2012").
Wang Y, Sharma RK, Falcone T, Goldberg J, Agarwal A. Importance of reactive oxygen species in the peritoneal fluid of

women with endometriosis or idiopathic infertility. Fertil Steril. 1997;68:826–30.

Van Langendonckt A, Casanas-Roux F, Donnez J. Oxidative stress and peritoneal endometriosis. Fertil Steril. 2002;77:861–70.

12 Victor VM, Rocha M, Banuls C, Alvarez A, de Pablo C, Sanchez-Serrano M, Gomez M, Hernandez-Mijares A. Induction of oxidative stress and human leukocyte/endothelial cell interactions in polycystic ovary syndrome patients with insulin resistance. J Clin Endocrinol Metab. 2011;96:3115–3122. ("Victor 2011").

13 Gonzalez F, Rote NS, Minium J, Kirwan JP. Reactive oxygen species-induced oxidative stress in the development of insulin resistance and hyperandrogenism in polycystic ovary syndrome. J Clin Endocrinol Metab. 2006;91:336–340.

Palacio JR, Iborra A, Ulcova-Gallova Z, Badia R, Martinez P. The presence of antibodies to oxidative modified proteins in serum from polycystic ovary syndrome patients. Clin Exp Immunol. 2006;144:217–222.

14 Victor 2011., Rajani 2012.

15 Patel SM, Nestler JE. Fertility in polycystic ovary syndrome. Endocrinol Metab Clin North Am. 2006;35:137–55.

Wood JR, Dumesic DA, Abbott DH, Strauss JF., III Molecular abnormalities in oocytes from women with polycystic ovary syndrome revealed by microarray analysis. J Clin Endocrinol Metab. 2007;92:705–13.

16 Wiener-Megnazi Z, Vardi L, Lissak A, Shnizer S, Reznick AZ, Ishai D, Lahav-Baratz S, Shiloh H, Koifman M, Dirnfeld M. Oxidative stress indices in follicular fluid as measured by the thermochemiluminescence assay correlate with outcome parameters in in vitro fertilization. Fertil Steril. 2004;82(Suppl 3):1171–1176.

de Bruin 2004, Eichenlaub 2011, premkumar 2012, Carbone 2003, Tatone 2006,

17 Wang LY, Wang DH, Zou XY, Xu CM. Mitochondrial functions on oocytes and preimplantation embryos. J Zhejiang Univ Sci B. 2009 Jul;10(7):483-92.

18 Shaum KM, Polotsky AJ.Nutrition and reproduction: is there evidence to support a "Fertility Diet" to improve mitochondrial function? Maturitas. 2013 Apr;74(4):309-12.

19 Showell MG, Brown J, Clarke J, Hart RJ. Antioxidants for female subfertility. Cochrane Database Syst Rev. 2013 Aug 5;8:CD007807.

20 E.g.: Ruder EH, Hartman TJ, Reindollar RH, Goldman MB. Female dietary antioxidant intake and time to pregnancy among

couples treated for unexplained infertility. Fertil Steril. 2013 Dec 17 [Epub ahead of print]. ("Ruder 2014").

21 Aydin Y, Ozatik O, Hassa H, Ulusoy D, Ogut S, Sahin F.Relationship between oxidative stress and clinical pregnancy in assisted reproductive technology treatment cycles. J Assist Reprod Genet. 2013 Jun;30(6):765-72.

22 Ruder 2014.

23 Chemineau P, Guillaume D, Migaud M, Thiéry JC, Pellicer-Rubio MT, Malpaux B. Seasonality of reproduction in mammals: intimate regulatory mechanisms and practical implications. Reprod Domest Anim. 2008 Jul;43 Suppl 2:40-7.

24 Brzezinski A, Seibel MM, Lynch HJ, Deng MH, Wurtman RJ. Melatonin in human preovulatory follicular fluid. J Clin Endocrinol Metab. 1987;64(4):865–867.
Ronnberg L, Kauppila A, Leppaluoto J, Martikainen H, Vakkuri O. Circadian and seasonal variation in human preovulatory follicular fluid melatonin concentration. J Clin Endocrinol Metab. 1990;71(2):492–496.

25 Nakamura Y, Tamura H, Takayama H, Kato H. Increased endogenous level of melatonin in preovulatory human follicles does not directly influence progesterone production. Fertil Steril. 2003 Oct;80(4):1012-6.

26 Tamura H, Takasaki A, Taketani T, Tanabe M, Kizuka F, Lee L, Tamura I, Maekawa R, Aasada H, Yamagata Y, Sugino N. The role of melatonin as an antioxidant in the follicle. J Ovarian Res. 2012 Jan 26;5:5. ("Tamura 2012").

27 Poeggeler B, Reiter RJ, Tan DX, Chen LD, Manchester LC. Melatonin, hydroxyl radical-mediated oxidative damage, and aging: a hypothesis. J Pineal Res. 1993;14(4):151–168.
Schindler AE, Christensen B, Henkel A, Oettel M, Moore C. High-dose pilot study with the novel progestogen dienogestin patients with endometriosis. Gynecol Endocrinol. 2006;22(1):9–17.

28 Reiter RJ, Tan DX, Manchester LC, Qi W. Biochemical reactivity of melatonin with reactive oxygen and nitrogen species: a review of the evidence. Cell Biochem Biophys. 2001;34(2):237–256.
Tan DX, Manchester LC, Reiter RJ, Plummer BF, Limson J, Weintraub ST, Qi W. Melatonin directly scavenges hydrogen peroxide: a potentially new metabolic pathway of melatonin biotransformation. Free Radic Biol Med. 2000;29(11):1177–1185. ("Tan 2000").

29 Tan 2000.

30 Sack RL, Lewy AJ, Erb DL, Vollmer WM, Singer CM. Human melatonin production decreases with age. J Pineal Res. 1986;3(4):379-88.

31 Tamura H, Takasaki A, Miwa I, Taniguchi K, Maekawa R, Asada H, Taketani T, Matsuoka A, Yamagata Y, Shimamura K. et al. Oxidative stress impairs oocyte quality and melatonin protects oocytes from free radical damage and improves fertilization rate. J Pineal Res. 2008;44(3):280–287 ("Tamura 2008").

32 Jahnke G, Marr M, Myers C, Wilson R, Travlos G, Price C. Maternal and developmental toxicity evaluation of melatonin administered orally to pregnant Sprague-Dawley rats. Toxicol Sci. 1999;50(2):271–279.

33 Ishizuka B, Kuribayashi Y, Murai K, Amemiya A, Itoh MT. The effect of melatonin on in vitro fertilization and embryo development in mice. J Pineal Res. 2000;28(1):48–51.

34 Papis K, Poleszczuk O, Wenta-Muchalska E, Modlinski JA. Melatonin effect on bovine embryo development in vitro in relation to oxygen concentration. J Pineal Res. 2007;43(4):321–326. Shi JM, Tian XZ, Zhou GB, Wang L, Gao C, Zhu SE, Zeng SM, Tian JH, Liu GS. Melatonin exists in porcine follicular fluid and improves in vitro maturation and parthenogenetic development of porcine oocytes. J Pineal Res. 2009;47(4):318–323.

35 Tamura 2012.

36 Tamura 2008; Tamura 2012.

37 Tamura 2012.

38 Interview with Dr. Tamura, published on September 15, 2010, http://www.news-medical.net/news/20100915/Hormone-melatonin-improves-egg-quality-in-IVF.aspx

39 Rizzo P, Raffone E, Benedetto V.Effect of the treatment with myo-inositol plus folic acid plus melatonin in comparison with a treatment with myo-inositol plus folic acid on oocyte quality and pregnancy outcome in IVF cycles. A prospective, clinical trial.Eur Rev Med Pharmacol Sci. 2010 Jun;14(6):555-61.

40 Woo MM, Tai CJ, Kang SK, Nathwani PS, Pang SF, Leung PC.Direct action of melatonin in human granulosa-luteal cells.J Clin Endocrinol Metab. 2001 Oct;86(10):4789-97.

41 Obayashi K, Saeki K, Iwamoto J, Okamoto N, Tomioka K, Nezu S, Ikada Y, Kurumatani N. Positive effect of daylight exposure on nocturnal urinary melatonin excretion in the elderly: a cross-sectional analysis of the HEIJO-KYO study. J Clin Endocrinol Metab. 2012 Nov;97(11):4166-73.

42 U.S. National Library of Medicine, National Institutes of Health, Medline Plus. *Melatonin.* 2011. Available at http://www.nlm.nih.gov/medlineplus/druginfo/natural/940.html

43 Natarajan 2010; Olson SE, Seidel GE., Jr Culture of in vitro-produced bovine embryos with vitamin E improves development in vitro and after transfer to recipients. Biol Reprod. 2000;62(2):248–252.

44 Tamura H, Takasaki A, Miwa I, Taniguchi K, Maekawa R, Asada H, Taketani T, Matsuoka A, Yamagata Y, Shimamura K, Morioka H, Ishikawa H, Reiter RJ, Sugino N. Oxidative stress impairs oocyte quality and melatonin protects oocytes from free radical damage and improves fertilization rate. J Pineal Res. 2008 Apr;44(3):280-7.

45 http://www.efsa.europa.eu/en/efsajournal/pub/640.htm

46 Mayo Clinic, 2012, Vitamin E Dosing. Available at http://www.mayoclinic.com/health/vitamin-e/NS_patient-vitamine/DSECTION=dosing

47 Colorado Center for Reproductive Medicine. Female Fertility Supplements. 2012.
http://www.colocrm.com/FertilitySupplements.aspx

48 Ruder EH, Hartman TJ, Reindollar RH, Goldman MB. Female dietary antioxidant intake and time to pregnancy among couples treated for unexplained infertility. Fertil Steril. 2013 Dec 17 [Epub ahead of print]. ("Ruder 2014").

49 Yeh J, Bowman MJ, Browne RW, Chen N. Reproductive aging results in a reconfigured ovarian antioxidant defense profile in rats. Fertil Steril. 2005 Oct;84 Suppl 2:1109-13;
Ruder 2014.

50 Luck MR, Jeyaseelan I, Scholes RA. Ascorbic acid and fertility. Biol Reprod. 1995 Feb;52(2):262-6;
Zreik TG, Kodaman PH, Jones EE, Olive DL, Behrman H. Identification and characterization of an ascorbic acid transporter in human granulosa-lutein cells. Mol Hum Reprod. 1999 Apr;5(4):299-302.

51 Tarín J, Ten J, Vendrell FJ, de Oliveira MN, Cano A. Effects of maternal ageing and dietary antioxidant supplementation on ovulation, fertilisation and embryo development in vitro in the mouse. Reprod Nutr Dev. 1998 Sep-Oct;38(5):499-508;
Tarín JJ, Pérez-Albalá S, Cano A. Oral antioxidants counteract the negative effects of female aging on oocyte quantity and quality in the mouse. Mol Reprod Dev. 2002 Mar;61(3):385-97;

Ozkaya MO, Nazıroğlu M. Multivitamin and mineral supplementation modulates oxidative stress and antioxidant vitamin levels in serum and follicular fluid of women undergoing in vitro fertilization. Fertil Steril. 2010 Nov;94(6):2465-6.

52 Ruder 2014.

53 Colorado Center for Reproductive Medicine. Female Fertility Supplements. 2012.
http://www.colocrm.com/FertilitySupplements.aspx

54 Bentov Y, Esfandiari N, Burstein E, Casper RF.The use of mitochondrial nutrients to improve the outcome of infertility treatment in older patients. Fertil Steril. 2010 Jan;93(1):272-5 ("Bentov 2010.")

55 Goraca A, Huk-Kolega H, Piechota A, Kleniewska P, Ciejka E, et al. (2011) Lipoic acid - biological activity and therapeutic potential. Pharmacol Rep 63: 849–858.

56 Packer L, Witt EH, Tritschler HJ: -Lipoic acid as a biological antioxidant. Free Radic Biol Med, 1995, 19, 227–250.

57 Arivazhagan P, Ramanathan K, Panneerselvam C: Effect of DL— lipoic acid on mitochondrial enzymes in aged rats. Chem Biol Interact, 2001, 138, 189–198.
Mc Carthy MF, Barroso-Aranda J, Contreras F: The "rejuvenatory" impact of lipoic acid on mitochondrial function in aging rats may reflect induction and activation of PPAR-coactivator-1. Med Hypotheses, 2009, 72, 29–33

58 Zembron-Lacny A, Slowinska-Lisowska M, Szygula Z, Witkowski K, Szyszka K. The comparison of antioxidant and hematological properties of N-acetylcysteine and alpha-lipoic acid in physically active males. Physiol Res Academ Sci Bohemoslov. 2009;58(6):855–861; Sun 2012. Zhang 2013

59 Talebi A, Zavareh S, Kashani MH, Lashgarbluki T, Karimi I.The effect of alpha lipoic acid on the developmental competence of mouse isolated preantral follicles. J Assist Reprod Genet. 2012 Feb;29(2):175-83.
Zhang H, Wu B, Liu H, Qiu M, Liu J, Zhang Y, Quan F. Improving development of cloned goat embryos by supplementing α-lipoic acid to oocyte in vitro maturation medium. Theriogenology. 2013 Aug;80(3):228-33.

60 Bentov Y, Yavorska T, Esfandiari N, Jurisicova A, Casper RF.The contribution of mitochondrial function to reproductive aging.J Assist Reprod Genet. 2011 Sep;28(9):773-83. ("Bentov 2011").

61 Bentov 2010.

62 Bentov 2013.

63 Masharani U, Gjerde C, Evans JL, Youngren JF, Goldfine ID. Effects of controlled-release alpha lipoic acid in lean, nondiabetic patients with polycystic ovary syndrome. J Diabetes Sci Technol. 2010 Mar 1;4(2):359-64.

64 Ghibu S, Richard C, Vergely C, Zeller M, Cottin Y, Rochette L: Antioxidant properties of an endogenous thiol: Alpha-lipoic acid, useful in the prevention of car- diovascular diseases. J Cardiovasc Pharmacol, 2009, 54, 391–398.

Shay KP, Moreau RF, Smith EJ, Smith AR, Hagen TM: Alpha-lipoic acid as a dietary supplement: Molecular mechanisms and therapeutic potential. Biochim Biophys Acta, 2009, 1790, 1149–1160.

Ziegler D, Hanefeld M, Ruhnau KJ, Hasche H, Lobisch M, Schutte K, Kerun G et al.: Treatment of symptomatic diabetic polyneuropathy with the antioxidant -lipoic acid: a 7-month multicenter randomized controled trial (ALADIN III study). Diabetes Care, 1999, 22, 1296–1301.

65 Ghibu S, Richard C, Vergely C, Zeller M, Cottin Y, Rochette L: Antioxidant properties of an endogenous thiol: Alpha-lipoic acid, useful in the prevention of cardiovascular diseases. J Cardiovasc Pharmacol, 2009, 54, 391–398.

Shay KP, Moreau RF, Smith EJ, Smith AR, Hagen TM: Alpha-lipoic acid as a dietary supplement: Molecular mechanisms and therapeutic potential. Biochim Biophys Acta, 2009, 1790, 1149–1160.

Ziegler D, Nowak H, Kempler P, Vargha P & Low PA. Treatment of symptomatic diabetic polyneuropathy with the antioxidant α-lipoic acid: a meta-analysis. Diabetic Medicine 2004 21 114–121.

66 Segermann J, Hotze A, Ulrich H, et al. Effect of alpha-lipoic acid on the peripheral conversion of thyroxine to triiodothyronine and on serum lipid-, protein- and glucose levels. Arzneimittelforschung. 1991;41:1294-1298.

67 Porasuphatana S, Suddee S, Nartnampong A, et al. Gylcemic and oxidative status of patients with type 2 diabetes mellitus following oral administration of alpha-lipoic acid: a randomized double-blinded placebo-controlled study. Asia Pac J Clin Nutr 2012;21(1):12–21.

Golbidi S, Badran M, Laher I. Diabetes and alpha lipoic Acid. Front Pharmacol. 2011;2:69.

68 Manning PJ, Sutherland WH, Williams SM, Walker RJ, Berry EA, De Jong SA, Ryalls AR. The effect of lipoic acid and vitamin E

therapies in individuals with the metabolic syndrome. Nutr Metab Cardiovasc Dis. 2013 Jun;23(6):543-9.

Wray DW, Nishiyama SK, Harris RA, Zhao J, McDaniel J, Fjeldstad AS, Witman MA, Ives SJ, Barrett-O'Keefe Z, Richardson RS. Acute reversal of endothelial dysfunction in the elderly after antioxidant consumption. Hypertension. 2012 Apr;59(4):818-24.

Ramos LF, Kane J, McMonagle E, Le P, Wu P, Shintani A, Ikizler TA, Himmelfarb J. Effects of combination tocopherols and alpha lipoic acid therapy on oxidative stress and inflammatory biomarkers in chronic kidney disease. J Ren Nutr. 2011 May;21(3):211-8.

69 Goraca A, Huk-Kolega H, Piechota A, Kleniewska P, Ciejka E, et al. (2011) Lipoic acid - biological activity and therapeutic potential. Pharmacol Rep 63: 849–858.

70 Hermann R, Niebch G, Borbe H.O, Fieger-Büschges H, Ruus P, Nowak H, Riethmüller-Winzen H et al.: Enanti- oselective pharmacokinetics and bioavailability of different racemic alpha-lipoic acid formulations in healthy volunteers. Eur J Clin Pharmacol Sci, 1996, 4, 167–174.)

71 Gleiter CH, Schug BS, Hermann R, Elze M, Blume HH, Gundert-Remy U: Influence of food intake on the bioa- vailability of thioctic acid enantiomers (letter). Eur J Clin Pharmacol, 1996, 50, 513–514

72 Atkuri KR, Mantovani JJ, Herzenberg LA, Herzenberg LA.N-Acetylcysteine—a safe antidote for cysteine/glutathione deficiency. Curr Opin Pharmacol. 2007 Aug;7(4):355-9. ("Atkuri 2007").

73 Dodd S, Dean O, Copolov DL, Malhi GS, Berk M.N-acetylcysteine for antioxidant therapy: pharmacology and clinical utility. Expert Opin Biol Ther. 2008 Dec;8(12):1955-62. Atkuri 2007.

74 Nasr A. Effect of N-acetyl-cysteine after ovarian drilling in clomiphene citrate-resistant PCOS women: a pilot study.Reprod Biomed Online. 2010 Mar;20(3):403-9. ("Nasr 2010").

75 Salehpour S, Sene AA, Saharkhiz N, Sohrabi MR, Moghimian F.N-Acetylcysteine as an adjuvant to clomiphene citrate for successful induction of ovulation in infertile patients with polycystic ovary syndrome.J Obstet Gynaecol Res. 2012 Sep;38(9):1182-6.

76 Kilic-Okman T, Kucuk M. N-acetyl-cysteine treatment for polycystic ovary syndrome. Int J Gynaecol Obstet 2004; 85: 296–297.

77 Liu J, Liu M, Ye X, Liu K, Huang J, Wang L, Ji G, Liu N, Tang X, Baltz JM, Keefe DL, Liu L.Delay in oocyte aging in mice by

the antioxidant N-acetyl-L-cysteine (NAC).Hum Reprod. 2012 May;27(5):1411-20. ("Liu 2012").

78 Liu L, Trimarchi JR, Smith PJ, Keefe DL. Mitochondrial dysfunction leads to telomere attrition and genomic instability. Aging Cell 2002; 1:40–46.
Liu L, Trimarchi JR, Navarro P, Blasco MA, Keefe DL. Oxidative stress contributes to arsenic-induced telomere attrition, chromosome instability, and apoptosis. J Biol Chem 2003;278:31998–32004.
Navarro PA, Liu L, Ferriani RA, Keefe DL. Arsenite induces aberrations in meiosis that can be prevented by coadministration of N-acetylcysteine in mice. Fertil Steril 2006;85 Suppl 1:1187 -1194
Huang J, Okuka M, McLean M, Keefe DL, Liu L. Telomere susceptibility to cigarette smoke-induced oxidative damage and chromosomal instability of mouse embryos in vitro. Free Radic Biol Med 2010;48:1663–1676.

79 Whitaker BD, Casey SJ, Taupier R. The effects of N-acetyl-L-cysteine supplementation on in vitro porcine oocyte maturation and subsequent fertilisation and embryonic development. Reprod Fertil Dev. 2012;24(8):1048-54.

80 Amin AF, Shaaban OM, Bediawy MA.N-acetyl cysteine for treatment of recurrent unexplained pregnancy loss. Reprod Biomed Online. 2008 Nov;17(5):722-6.

81 Nasr 2010.

82 Dodd 2008, Atkuri 2007

83 Lynch RM, Robertson R. Anaphylactoid reactions to intravenous N-acetylcysteine: a prospective case controlled study.Accid Emerg Nurs. 2004 Jan;12(1):10-5.

84 Appelboam AV, Dargan PI, Knighton J. Fatal anaphylactoid reaction to N-acetylcysteine: caution in patients with asthma. Emerg Med J. 2002 Nov;19(6):594-5.

85 Liu 2012; Nasr 2010.

86 Lim J, Luderer U. Oxidative damage increases and antioxidant gene expression decreases with aging in the mouse ovary. Biol Reprod. 2011 Apr;84(4):775-82; Liu 2012.

Chapter 8: Restoring Ovulation with Myo-Inositol

1 Mitchell Bebel Stargrove, Jonathan Treasure, Dwight L. McKee. Herb, Nutrient, and Drug Interactions: Clinical Implications and Therapeutic Strategies, Health Sciences, 2008, p. 765.

2 Chiu TT, Rogers MS, Law EL, Briton-Jones CM, Cheung LP, Haines CJ.Follicular fluid and serum concentrations of

myo-inositol in patients undergoing IVF: relationship with oocyte quality.Hum Reprod. 2002 Jun;17(6):1591-6. ("Chiu 2002").

3 Downes, C.P. (1989) The cellular function of myo-inositol. Biochem. Soc. Trans., 17, 259–268; Downes, C.P. and Macphee, C.H. (1990) Review: myo-inositol metabolites as cellular signals. Eur. J. Biochem., 193, 1–18.

4 Papaleo E, Unfer V, Baillargeon JP, Fusi F, Occhi F, De Santis L.Myo-inositol may improve oocyte quality in intracytoplasmic sperm injection cycles. A prospective, controlled, randomized trial. Fertil Steril. 2009 May;91(5):1750-4; ("Papaleo 2009").
Genazzani AD, Lanzoni C, Ricchieri F, Jasonni VM. Myo-inositol administration positively affects hyperinsulinemia and hormonal parameters in overweight patients with polycystic ovary syndrome. Gynecol Endocrinol. 2008 Mar;24(3):139-44. ("Genazzani 2008").

5 Baptiste CG, Battista MC, Trottier A, Baillargeon JP. Insulin and hyperandrogenism in women with polycystic ovary syndrome. J Steroid Biochem Mol Biol. 2010 Oct;122(1-3):42-52.
Filicori M, Flamigni C, Campaniello E, Meriggiola MC, Michelacci L, Valdiserri A, Ferrari P. Polycystic ovary syndrome: abnormalities and management with pulsatile gonadotropin-releasing hormone and gonadotropin-releasing hormone analogs. Am J Obstet Gynecol. 1990 Nov;163(5 Pt 2):1737-42.

6 Hasegawa I, Murakawa H, Suzuki M, Yamamoto Y, Kurabayashi T, Tanaka K. Effect of troglitazone on endocrine and ovulatory performance in women with insulin resistance-related polycystic ovary syndrome. Fertil Steril. 1999 Feb;71(2):323-7.
Ng EH, Wat NM, Ho PC. Effects of metformin on ovulation rate, hormonal and metabolic profiles in women with clomiphene-resistant polycystic ovaries: a randomized, double-blinded placebo-controlled trial. Hum Reprod. 2001 Aug;16(8):1625-31.
Lord JM, Flight IH, Norman RJ. Metformin in polycystic ovary syndrome: systematic review and meta-analysis. BMJ. 2003 Oct 25;327(7421):951-3.

7 Fleming R, Hopkinson ZE, Wallace AM, Greer IA, Sattar N. Ovarian function and metabolic factors in women with oligomenorrhea treated with metformin in a randomized double blind placebo-controlled trial. J Clin Endocrinol Metab 2002;87: 569-74.

8 Papaleo E, Unfer V, Baillargeon JP, De Santis L, Fusi F, Brigante C, Marelli G, Cino I, Redaelli A, Ferrari A. Myo-inositol in patients with polycystic ovary syndrome: a novel method for ovulation induction. Gynecol Endocrinol. 2007 Dec;23(12):700-3.

9 Genazzani 2008.
10 Costantino D, Minozzi G, Minozzi E, Guaraldi C.Metabolic and hormonal effects of myo-inositol in women with polycystic ovary syndrome: a double-blind trial.Eur Rev Med Pharmacol Sci. 2009 Mar-Apr;13(2):105-10.
11 Papaleo 2009
12 Ciotta L, Stracquadanio M, Pagano I, Carbonaro A, Palumbo M, Gulino F.Effects of myo-inositol supplementation on oocyte's quality in PCOS patients: a double blind trial.Eur Rev Med Pharmacol Sci. 2011 May;15(5):509-14.
13 Unfer V, Carlomagno G, Rizzo P, Raffone E, Roseff S. Myo-inositol rather than D-chiro-inositol is able to improve oocyte quality in intracytoplasmic sperm injection cycles. A prospective, controlled, randomized trial. Eur Rev Med Pharmacol Sci. 2011 Apr;15(4):452-7.
14 Berridge, M.J. Inositol triphosphate and calcium signalling. Nature, 1993, 361, 315–325; Fujiwara, T., Nakada, K., Shirakawa, H. and Miyazaki, S. (Determination of inositol trisphosphate-induced calcium release mechanism during maturation of hamster oocytes. Dev. Biol. 1993, 156, 69–79; Downes 1989
15 Baillargeon JP, Diamanti-Kandarakis E, Ostlund RE Jr, Apridonidze T, Iuorno MJ, Nestler JE. Altered D-chiro-inositol urinary clearance in women with polycystic ovary syndrome. Diabetes Care. 2006 Feb;29(2):300-5; Constantino 2009.
16 Chiu TT, Rogers MS, Briton-Jones C, Haines C. Effects of myo-inositol on the in-vitro maturation and subsequent development of mouse oocytes. Hum Reprod. 2003 Feb;18(2):408-16.
17 D'Anna R, Di Benedetto V, Rizzo P, Raffone E, Interdonato ML, Corrado F, Di Benedetto A. Myo-inositol may prevent gestational diabetes in PCOS women. Gynecol Endocrinol. 2012 Jun;28(6):440-2
18 Lisi F, Carfagna P, Oliva MM, Rago R, Lisi R, Poverini R, Manna C, Vaquero E, Caserta D, Raparelli V, Marci R, Moscarini M.Pretreatment with myo-inositol in non polycystic ovary syndrome patients undergoing multiple follicular stimulation for IVF: a pilot study. Reprod Biol Endocrinol. 2012 Jul 23;10:52. ("Lisi 2012").
19 Craig LB, Ke RW, Kutteh WH.Increased prevalence of insulin resistance in women with a history of recurrent pregnancy loss. Fertil Steril. 2002 Sep;78(3):487-90. ("Craig 2002").
20 Craig 2002.
21 Hong Y, Xie QX, Chen CY, Yang C, Li YZ, Chen DM, Xie MQ.Insulin resistance in first-trimester pregnant women

with pre-pregnant glucose tolerance and history of recurrent spontaneous abortion.J Biol Regul Homeost Agents. 2013 Jan-Mar;27(1):225-31.

22 Lisi 2012; Carlomagno G, Unfer V.Inositol safety: clinical evidences. Eur Rev Med Pharmacol Sci. 2011 Aug;15(8):931-6.

23 Isabella R, Raffone E. Does ovary need D-chiro-inositol? J Ovarian Res. 2012 May 15;5(1):14. ("Isabella 2012").

24 Galletta M, Grasso S, Vaiarelli A, Roseff SJ. Bye-bye chiro-inositol - myo-inositol: true progress in the treatment of polycystic ovary syndrome and ovulation induction. Eur Rev Med Pharmacol Sci. 2011 Oct;15(10):1212-4.

25 Isabella 2012

26 Carlomagno G, Unfer V, Roseff S.The D-chiro-inositol paradox in the ovary.Fertil Steril. 2011 Jun 30;95(8):2515-6.

Chapter 9: DHEA for Diminished Ovarian Reserve

1 Fouany MR, Sharara FI. Is there a role for DHEA supplementation in women with diminished ovarian reserve? J Assist Reprod Genet. 2013 Sep;30(9):1239-44.

2 http://www.centerforhumanreprod.com/dhea.html

3 Wiser A, Gonen O, Ghetler Y, Shavit T, Berkovitz A, Shulman A. Addition of dehydroepiandrosterone (DHEA) for poor-responder patients before and during IVF treatment improves the pregnancy rate: a randomized prospective study. Hum Reprod. 2010 Oct;25(10):2496-500 ("Wiser 2010").

4 Harper AJ, Buster JE, Casson PR. Changes in adrenocortical function with aging and therapeutic implications. Semin Reprod Endocrinol. 1999;17(4):327-38.

5 Arlt W. Dehydroepiandrosterone and aging. Best Pract Res Clin Endocrinol 2004;18:363.

6 Casson PR, Lindsay MS, Pisarska MD, Carson SA, Buster JE. Dehydroepiandrosterone supplementation augments ovarian stimulation in poor responders: a case series. Hum Reprod 2000;15:2129-2132.

7 Barad DH, et al, Update on the use of dehydroepiandrosterone supplementation among women with diminished ovarian reserve. J Assist Reprod Genet 2007;24(12):629-34.

8 http://www.centerforhumanreprod.com/dhea.html, interview with CBS News.

9 http://www.centerforhumanreprod.com/dhea.html, interview with CBS News.

10 Gleicher N, Barad DH. Dehydroepiandrosterone (DHEA) supplementation in diminished ovarian reserve (DOR). Reprod Biol Endocrinol. 2011 May 17;9:67 ("Gleicher 2011").

11 Gleicher 2011

12 Ulug U, Ben-Shlomo I, Turan E, Erden HF, Akman MA, Bahceci M. Conception rates following assisted reproduction in poor responder patients: a retrospective study in 300 consecutive cycles. Reprod Biomed Online 2003;6:439-443;
Frattarelli JL, Hill MJ, McWilliams GD, Miller KA, Bergh PA, Scott RT Jr.. A luteal estradiol protocol for expected poor-responders improves embryo number and quality. Fertil Steril 2008;89:1118-1122;
Schmidt DW, Bremner T, Orris JJ, Maier DB, Benadiva CA, Nulsen JC . A randomized prospective study of microdose leuprolide versus ganirelix in in vitro fertilization cycles for poor responders. Fertil Steril 2005;83:1568-1571.

13 Barad DH and Gleicher N, Effects of dehydroepiandrosterone on oocyte and embryo yields, embryo grade and cell number in IVF. Hum Reprod 2006;21(11):2845-9.

14 Barad DH, et al, Update on the use of dehydroepiandrosterone supplementation among women with diminished ovarian reserve. J Assist Reprod Genet 2007;24(12):629-34.

15 Mamas L, Mamas E. Dehydroepiandrosterone supplementation in assisted reproduction: rationale and results. Curr Opin Obstet Gynecol. 2009 Aug;21(4):306-8;
Hyman JH, Margalioth EJ, Rabinowitz R, Tsafrir A, Gal M, Alerhand S, Algur N, Eldar-Geva T. DHEA supplementation may improve IVF outcome in poor responders: a proposed mechanism. Eur J Obstet Gynecol Reprod Biol. 2013 May;168(1):49-53 ("Hyman 2013").

16 Sönmezer M, Ozmen B, Cil AP, Ozkavukçu S, Taşçi T, Olmuş H, Atabekoğlu CS. Dehydroepiandrosterone supplementation improves ovarian response and cycle outcome in poor responders. Reprod Biomed Online. 2009 Oct;19(4):508-13.

17 Wiser 2010

18 Yeung TW, Li RH, Lee VC, Ho PC, Ng EH. A randomized double-blinded placebo-controlled trial on the effect of dehydroepiandrosterone for 16 weeks on ovarian response markers in women with primary ovarian insufficiency. J Clin Endocrinol Metab. 2013 Jan;98(1):380-8.

19 Bedaiwy MA, Ryan E, Shaaban O, Claessens EA, Blanco-Mejia S, Casper RF: Follicular conditioning with dehydroepiandrosterone

co-treatment improves IUI outcome in clomiphene citrate patients. 55th Annual Meeting of the Canadian Fertility and Andrology Society, Montreal, Canada, November 18-21, 2009.

20 Fusi FM, Ferrario M, Bosisio C, Arnoldi M, Zanga L. DHEA supplementation positively affects spontaneous pregnancies in women with diminished ovarian function. Gynecol Endocrinol. 2013 Oct;29(10):940-3 ("Fusi 2013").

21 Barad 2007.

22 Barad 2007; Fusi 2013.

23 Gleicher N, et al, Miscarriage rates after dehydroepiandrosterone (DHEA) supplementation in women with diminished ovarian reserve: a case control study. Reprod Biol Endocrinol 2009;7(7):108 ("Gleicher 2009").

24 Levi AJ, Raynault MF, Bergh PA, Drews MR, Miller BT, Scott RT Jr: Reproductive outcome in patients with diminished ovarian reserve. Fertil Steril 2001, 76:666-669.

25 Gleicher N, et al, Dehydroepiandrosterone (DHEA) reduces embryo aneuploidy: direct evidence from preimplantation genetic screening (PGS). Reprod Biol Endocrinol 2010;10(8):140 ("Gleicher 2010a")
Gleicher 2009.

26 Gleicher 2010a.

27 Gleicher 2010a.

28 Casson PR, Lindsay MS, Pisarska MD, Carson SA, Buster JE. Dehydroepiandrosterone supplementation augments ovarian stimulation in poor responders: a case series. Hum Reprod 2002; 15:2129–2132.

29 Sen A, Hammes SR: Granulosa cell-specific androgen receptors are critical regulators of development and function. Mol Endocrinol 2010, 24:1393-1403.

30 Hyman 2013.

31 Gleicher 2011.

32 Gleicher 2011.

33 Bentov Y, Casper RF. The aging oocyte—can mitochondrial function be improved? Fertil Steril. 2013 Jan;99(1):18-22.

34 Yakin K, Urman B. DHEA as a miracle drug in the treatment of poor responders; hype or hope? Hum Reprod. 2011 Aug;26(8):1941-4 ("Yakin 2011").

35 Urman B, Yakin K. DHEA for poor responders: can treatment be justified in the absence of evidence? Reprod Biomed Online. 2012 Aug;25(2):103-7.

36 Gleicher 2011.

37 Gleicher N, Barad DH. Misplaced obsession with prospectively randomized studies. Reprod Biomed Online. 2010 Oct;21(4):440-3 ("Gleicher 2010b").

38 Yakin 2011.

39 Wald NJ. Commentary: a brief history of folic acid in the prevention of neural tube defects. Int J Epidemiol. 2011 Oct;40(5):1154-6;
Schorah C. Commentary: from controversy and procrastination to primary prevention. Int J Epidemiol. 2011 Oct;40(5):1156-8.

40 Li L, Ferin M, Sauer MV, Lobo RA. Dehydroepiandrosterone in follicular fluid is produced locally, and levels correlate negatively with in vitro fertilization outcomes. Fertil Steril. 2011 Apr;95(5):1830-2.

41 Gleicher 2010a.

42 Yilmaz N, Uygur D, Inal H, Gorkem U, Cicek N, Mollamahmutoglu L. Dehydroepiandrosterone supplementation improves predictive markers for diminished ovarian reserve: serum AMH, inhibin B and antral follicle count. Eur J Obstet Gynecol Reprod Biol. 2013 Jul;169(2):257-60; Fouany 2013.

43 Gleicher 2011.

44 Yakin 2011.

45 Gleicher 2011

46 Gleicher 2011.

47 Wiser 2010.

48 Panjari M, Bell RJ, Jane F, Adams J, Morrow C, Davis SR: The safety of 52 weeks of oral DHEA therapy for postmenopausal women. Maturitas 2009, 63:240-245.

49 Parasrampuria J, Schwartz K, Petesch R. Quality control of dehydroepiandrosterone dietary supplement products. JAMA. 1998 Nov 11;280(18):1565.

50 Casson PR, Straughn AB, Umstot ES, Abraham GE, Carson SA, Buster JE. Delivery of dehydroepiandrosterone to premenopausal women: effects of micronization and nonoral administration. Am J Obstet Gynecol. 1996 Feb;174(2):649-53.

51 Gleicher 2011; Wiser 2010.

52 Intervew with Dr. Gleicher, published in ObGyn News 09/01/06.

Chapter 10: Supplements That May Do More Harm Than Good

1 http://www.pycnogenol.com/science/research-library/

2 Blank S, Bantleon FI, McIntyre M, Ollert M, Spillner E. The major royal jelly proteins 8 and 9 (Api m 11) are glycosylated

components of Apis mellifera venom with allergenic potential beyond carbohydrate-based reactivity. Clin Exp Allergy. 2012 Jun;42(6):976-85.

3 Morita H, Ikeda T, Kajita K, Fujioka K, Mori I, Okada H, Uno Y, Ishizuka T. Effect of royal jelly ingestion for six months on healthy volunteers. Nutr J. 2012 Sep 21;11:77.

4 Battaglia C, Salvatori M, Maxia N, Petraglia F, Facchinetti F, Volpe A. Adjuvant L-arginine treatment for in-vitro fertilization in poor responder patients. Hum Reprod. 1999 Jul;14(7):1690-7. ("Battaglia 1999").

5 Battaglia 1999.

6 Keay, S.D., Liversedge, N.H., Mathur, R.S. and Jenkins, J.M. Assisted conception following poor ovarian response to gonadotrophin stimulation. Br. J. Obstet. Gynecol. 1997,104, 521–527; Tanbo T, Abyholm T, Bjøro T, Dale PO. Ovarian stimulation in previous failures from in-vitro fertilization: distinction of two groups of poor responders. Hum Reprod. 1990 Oct;5(7):811-5.

7 Battaglia 1999.

8 Battaglia C, Regnani G, Marsella T, Facchinetti F, Volpe A, Venturoli S, Flamigni C. Adjuvant L-arginine treatment in controlled ovarian hyperstimulation: a double-blind, randomized study.Hum Reprod. 2002 Mar;17(3):659-65.

9 Agarwal A, Gupta S, Sekhon L, Shah R. Redox considerations in female reproductive function and assisted reproduction: from molecular mechanisms to health implications. Antioxid Redox Signal. 2008 Aug;10(8):1375-403.

10 Bódis J, Várnagy A, Sulyok E, Kovács GL, Martens-Lobenhoffer J, Bode-Böger SM.Negative association of L-arginine methylation products with oocyte numbers. Hum Reprod. 2010 Dec;25(12):3095-100. doi: 10.1093/humrep/deq257. Epub 2010 Sep 24.

11 Lee TH, Wu MY, Chen MJ, Chao KH, Ho HN, Yang YS. Nitric oxide is associated with poor embryo quality and pregnancy outcome in in vitro fertilization cycles. Fertil Steril. 2004 Jul;82(1):126-31.

Chapter 11: The Egg Quality Diet

1 Hjollund NHI, Jensen TK, Bonde JPE, Henriksen NE, Andersson AM, Skakkebaek NE. Is glycosilated haemoglobin a marker of fertility? A follow-up study of first-pregnancy planners. Hum Reprod. 1999;14:1478–1482 ("Hjolland 1999").

2 Hjolland 1999.

3 Chavarro JE, Rich-Edwards JW, Rosner BA, Willett WC. A prospective study of dietary carbohydrate quantity and quality

in relation to risk of ovulatory infertility. Eur J Clin Nutr. 2009 Jan;63(1):78-86 ("Chavarro 2009a").

4 Dumesic DA, Abbott DH. Implications of polycystic ovary syndrome on oocyte development. Semin Reprod Med. 2008 Jan;26(1):53-61.
Heijnen EMEW, Eijkemans MJC, Hughes EG, et al. A meta-analysis of outcomes of conventional IVF in women with polycstic ovary syndrome. Human Reprod Update. 2006;12:13–21.
Sengoku K, Tamate K, Takuma N, et al. The chromosomal normality of unfertilized oocytes from patients with polycystic ovarian syndrome. Hum Reprod. 1997;12:474–477.
Ludwig M, Finas DF, Al-Hasani S, et al. Oocyte quality and treatment outcome in intracytoplasmic sperm injection cycles of polycystic ovarian syndrome patients. Hum Reprod. 1999;14:354–358.

5 Dunaif A, Drug insight: insulin-sensitizing drugs in the treatment of polycystic ovary syndrome—a reappraisal. Nat Clin Pract Endocrinol Metab. 2008; 4:272–283
Palomba S, Falbo A, Zullo F, Orio F Jr. Evidence-based and potential benefits of metformin in the polycystic ovary syndrome: a comprehensive review. Endocr Rev. 2009; 30:1–50
Practice Committee of American Society for Reproductive Medicine. Use of insulin-sensitizing agents in the treatment of polycystic ovary syndrome. Fertil Steril. 2008; 90:S69–S73
Nestler JE, Metformin for the treatment of the polycystic ovary syndrome. N Engl J Med. 2008; 358:47–54

6 Ohgi S, Nakagawa K, Kojima R, Ito M, Horikawa T, Saito H. Insulin resistance in oligomenorrheic infertile women with non-polycystic ovary syndrome. Fertil Steril. 2008 Aug;90(2):373-7.

7 Diamanti-Kandarakis E, Dunaif A. Insulin resistance and the polycystic ovary syndrome revisited: an update on mechanisms and implications. Endocr Rev. 2012 Dec;33(6):981-1030 ("Diamanti-Kandarakis 2012").

8 Dumesic DA, Abbott DH. Implications of polycystic ovary syndrome on oocyte development. Semin Reprod Med. 2008 Jan;26(1):53-61.

9 Hjollund 1999; Jinno 2011; Chavarro 2009a

10 Azziz R, Ehrmann D, Legro RS, Whitcomb RW, Hanley R, Fereshetian AG, et al. Troglitazone improves ovulation and hirsutism in the polycystic ovary syndrome: A multicenter, double blind, placebo-controlled trial. J Clin Endocrinol Metab. 2001;86:1626–1632 ("Azziz 2001");

Brettenthaler N, De Geyter C, Huber PR, Keller U. Effect of the insulin sensitizer pioglitazone on insulin resistance, hyperandrogenism, and ovulatory dysfunction in women with polycystic ovary syndrome. J Clin Endocrinol Metab. 2004;89:3835–3840 ("Brettenthaler 2004");
Hjollund 1999.

11 Jinno 2011.

12 Jinno 2011.

13 Tatone C, Amicarelli F, Carbone MC, Monteleone P, Caserta D, Marci R, Artini PG, Piomboni P, Focarelli R. Cellular and molecular aspects of ovarian follicle ageing. Hum Reprod Update. 2008 Mar-Apr;14(2):131-42.

14 Wang Q, Moley KH. Maternal diabetes and oocyte quality. Mitochondrion. 2010 Aug;10(5):403-10 ("Wang 2010").

15 Craig LB, Ke RW, Kutteh WH. Increased prevalence of insulin resistance in women with a history of recurrent pregnancy loss. Fertil Steril. 2002 Sep;78(3):487-90.

16 Chakraborty P, Goswami SK, Rajani S, Sharma S, Kabir SN, Chakravarty B, Jana K. Recurrent pregnancy loss in polycystic ovary syndrome: role of hyperhomocysteinemia and insulin resistance. PLoS One. 2013 May 21;8(5):e64446;
Tian L, Shen H, Lu Q, Norman RJ, Wang J. Insulin resistance increases the risk of spontaneous abortion after assisted reproduction technology treatment. J Clin Endocrinol Metab. 2007 Apr;92(4):1430-3.

17 Hjolland 1999.

18 Azziz 2001; Brettenthaler 2004, Hjolland 1999

19 Brand-Miller JC. Glycemic load and chronic disease. Nutr Rev. 2003 May;61(5 Pt 2):S49-55.

20 Harvard Health Publications, Harvard Medical School, Glycemic Index and Glycemic Load for 100+ foods.

21 Melanson KJ, Zukley L, Lowndes J, Nguyen V, Angelopoulos TJ, Rippe JM. Effects of high-fructose corn syrup and sucrose consumption on circulating glucose, insulin, leptin, and ghrelin and on appetite in normal-weight women. Nutrition. 2007;23:103–112.
Stanhope KL, Griffen SC, Bair BR, Swarbrick MM, Keim NL, Havel PJ. Twenty-four-hour endocrine and metabolic profiles following consumption of high-fructose corn syrup-, sucrose-, fructose-, and glucose-sweetened beverages with meals. Am J Clin Nutr. 2008;87:1194–1203

22 Dekker MJ, Su Q, Baker C, Rutledge AC, Adeli K. Fructose: a highly lipogenic nutrient implicated in insulin resistance, hepatic

steatosis, and the metabolic syndrome. Am J Physiol Endocrinol Metab. 2010 Nov;299(5):E685-94.

23 Stanhope KL, Schwarz JM, Keim NL, Griffen SC, Bremer AA, Graham JL, Hatcher B, Cox CL, Dyachenko A, Zhang W, McGahan JP, Seibert A, Krauss RM, Chiu S, Schaefer EJ, Ai M, Otokozawa S, Nakajima K, Nakano T, Beysen C, Hellerstein MK, Berglund L, Havel PJ. Consuming fructose-sweetened, not glucose-sweetened, beverages increases visceral adiposity and lipids and decreases insulin sensitivity in overweight/obese humans. J Clin Invest. 2009 May;119(5):1322-34

24 Chavarro JE, Rich-Edwards JW, Rosner BA, Willett WC. Dietary fatty acid intakes and the risk of ovulatory infertility. Am J Clin Nutr. 2007;85:231–237

25 Saravanan N, Haseeb A, Ehtesham NZ, Ghafoorunissa. Differential effects of dietary saturated and trans-fatty acids on expression of genes associated with insulin sensitivity in rat adipose tissue. Eur J Endocrinol 2005;153:159–65.

26 Glueck CJ, Moreira A, Goldenberg N, Sieve L, Wang P. Pioglitazone and metformin in obese women with polycystic ovary syndrome not optimally responsive to metformin. Hum Reprod 2003;18:1618–25

Ghazeeri G, Kutteh WH, Bryer-Ash M, Haas DA, Ke RW. Effect of rosiglitazone on spontaneous and clomiphene citrate-induced ovulation in women with polycystic ovary syndrome. Fertil Steril 2003;79:562–6.

Cataldo NA, Abbasi F, McLaughlin TL, et al. Metabolic and ovarian effects of rosiglitazone treatment for 12 weeks in insulin-resistant women with polycystic ovary syndrome. Hum Reprod 2006;21:109–20.

27 Vujkovic M, de Vries JH, Lindemans J, Macklon NS, van der Spek PJ, Steegers EA, Steegers-Theunissen RP. The preconception Mediterranean dietary pattern in couples undergoing in vitro fertilization/intracytoplasmic sperm injection treatment increases the chance of pregnancy.Fertil Steril. 2010 Nov;94(6):2096-101 ("Vujkovic 2010").

28 Ebisch IM, Peters WH, Thomas CM, Wetzels AM, Peer PG, Steegers-Theunissen RP. Homocysteine, glutathione and related thiols affect fertility parameters in the (sub)fertile couple.Hum Reprod. 2006 Jul;21(7):1725-33.

29 Chakrabarty P, Goswami SK, Rajani S, Sharma S, Kabir SN, Chakravarty B, Jana K. Recurrent pregnancy loss in polycystic

ovary syndrome: role of hyperhomocysteinemia and insulin resistance. PLoS One. 2013 May 21;8(5):e64446; Wouters MG, Boers GH, Blom HJ, Trijbels FJ, Thomas CM, Borm GF, Steegers-Theunissen RP, Eskes TK. Hyperhomocysteinemia: a risk factor in women with unexplained recurrent early pregnancy loss. Fertil Steril. 1993 Nov;60(5):820-5.

30 Ronnenberg AG, Venners SA, Xu X, Chen C, Wang L, Guang W, Huang A, Wang X. Preconception B-vitamin and homocysteine status, conception, and early pregnancy loss.Am J Epidemiol. 2007 Aug 1;166(3):304-12.

31 Pawlak R, Parrott SJ, Raj S, Cullum-Dugan D, Lucus D. How prevalent is vitamin B(12) deficiency among vegetarians?Nutr Rev. 2013 Feb;71(2):110-7.

32 Twigt JM, Bolhuis ME, Steegers EA, Hammiche F, van Inzen WG, Laven JS, Steegers-Theunissen RP.The preconception diet is associated with the chance of ongoing pregnancy in women undergoing IVF/ICSI treatment. Hum Reprod. 2012 Aug;27(8):2526-31.

33 Vujkovic 2010

34 Hammiche F, Vujkovic M, Wijburg W, de Vries JH, Macklon NS, Laven JS, Steegers-Theunissen RP. Increased preconception omega-3 polyunsaturated fatty acid intake improves embryo morphology. Fertil Steril. 2011 Apr;95(5):1820-3.

35 Chilton, F., Win the War Within, Rodale, 2006.

36 Shaaker M, Rahimipour A, Nouri M, Khanaki K, Darabi M, Farzadi L, Shahnazi V, Mehdizadeh A. Fatty acid composition of human follicular fluid phospholipids and fertilization rate in assisted reproductive techniques. Iran Biomed J. 2012;16(3):162-8.

37 http://www.fda.gov/food/resourcesforyou/consumers/ucm110591. htm

38 Eggert J, Theobald H, Engfeldt P. Effects of alcohol consumption on female fertility during an 18-year period. Fertil Steril. 2004 Feb;81(2):379-83.

39 Juhl M, Nyboe Andersen AM, Grønbaek M, Olsen J. Moderate alcohol consumption and waiting time to pregnancy. Hum Reprod. 2001 Dec;16(12):2705-9; Jensen TK, Hjollund NH, Henriksen TB, Scheike T, Kolstad H, Giwercman A, Ernst E, Bonde JP, Skakkebaek NE, Olsen J. Does moderate alcohol consumption affect fertility? Follow up study among couples planning first pregnancy. BMJ. 1998 Aug 22;317(7157):505-10 ("Jensen 1998a");

Jensen TK, Henriksen TB, Hjollund NH, Scheike T, Kolstad H, Giwercman A, Ernst E, Bonde JP, Skakkebaek NE, Olsen J. Caffeine intake and fecundability: a follow-up study among 430 Danish couples planning their first pregnancy. Reprod Toxicol. 1998 May-Jun;12(3):289-95 ("Jensen 1998b").

40 Tolstrup JS, Kjaer SK, Holst C, Sharif H, Munk C, Osler M, Schmidt L, Andersen AM, Grønbaek M. Alcohol use as predictor for infertility in a representative population of Danish women. Acta Obstet Gynecol Scand. 2003 Aug;82(8):744-9.

41 Jensen 1998a

42 Grodstein F, Goldman MB, Cramer DW. Infertility in women and moderate alcohol use. Am J Public Health. 1994 Sep;84(9):1429-32; Chavarro JE, Rich-Edwards JW, Rosner BA, Willett WC. Caffeinated and alcoholic beverage intake in relation to ovulatory disorder infertility. Epidemiology. 2009 May;20(3):374-81.

43 Klonoff-Cohen H, Lam-Kruglick P, Gonzalez C. Effects of maternal and paternal alcohol consumption on the success rates of in vitro fertilization and gamete intrafallopian transfer. Fertil Steril. 2003 Feb;79(2):330-9.

44 Rossi BV, Berry KF, Hornstein MD, Cramer DW, Ehrlich S, Missmer SA. Effect of alcohol consumption on in vitro fertilization. Obstet Gynecol. 2011 Jan;117(1):136-42.

45 Hassan MA, Killick SR. Negative lifestyle is associated with a significant reduction in fecundity. Fertil Steril. 2004 Feb;81(2):384-92.

46 Huang H, Hansen KR, Factor-Litvak P, Carson SA, Guzick DS, Santoro N, Diamond MP, Eisenberg E, Zhang H; National Institute of Child Health and Human Development Cooperative Reproductive Medicine Network. Predictors of pregnancy and live birth after insemination in couples with unexplained or male-factor infertility. Fertil Steril. 2012 Apr;97(4):959-67.

47 Al-Saleh I, El-Doush I, Grisellhi B, Coskun S. The effect of caffeine consumption on the success rate of pregnancy as well various performance parameters of in-vitro fertilization treatment. Med Sci Monit. 2010 Dec;16(12):CR598-605.

Chapter 12: The Other Half of the Equation: Sperm Quality

1 Esteves SC, Agarwal A. Novel concepts in male infertility. Int Braz J Urol. 2011 Jan-Feb;37(1):5-15.

2 Kumar K, Deka D, Singh A, Mitra DK, Vanitha BR, Dada R. Predictive value of DNA integrity analysis in idiopathic recurrent

pregnancy loss following spontaneous conception. J Assist Reprod Genet. 2012 Sep;29(9):861-7.

3 Siddighi S, Chan CA, Patton WC, Jacobson JD, Chan PJ: Male age and sperm necrosis in assisted reproductive technologies. Urol Int. 2007; 9: 231-4 ("Siddighi 2007").

4 Singh NP, Muller CH, Berger RE. Effects of age on DNA double-strand breaks and apoptosis in human sperm. Fertil Steril. 2003 Dec;80(6):1420-30;
Wyrobek AJ, Eskenazi B, Young S, Arnheim N, Tiemann-Boege I, Jabs EW, Glaser RL, Pearson FS, Evenson D. Advancing age has differential effects on DNA damage, chromatin integrity, gene mutations, and aneuploidies in sperm. Proc Natl Acad Sci U S A. 2006 Jun 20;103(25):9601-6;
Schmid TE, Eskenazi B, Baumgartner A, Marchetti F, Young S, Weldon R, Anderson D, Wyrobek AJ. The effects of male age on sperm DNA damage in healthy non-smokers. Hum Reprod. 2007 Jan;22(1):180-7.

5 Moskovtsev SI, Willis J, Mullen JB: Age-related decline in sperm deoxyribonucleic acid integrity in patients evaluated for male infertility. Fertil Steril. 2006; 85: 496-9.

6 Wyrobek AJ, Aardema M, Eichenlaub-Ritter U, Ferguson L, Marchetti F: Mechanisms and targets involved in maternal and paternal age effects on numerical aneuploidy. Environ Mol Mutagen. 1996; 28: 254-64.

7 Hultman CM; Sandin S; Levine SZ; Lichtenstein P; Reichenberg A: Advancing paternal age and risk of autism: new evidence from a population-based study and a meta-analysis of epidemiological studies. Mol Psychiatry 2011; 16:1203–1212

8 Robinson L, Gallos ID, Conner SJ, Rajkhowa M, Miller D, Lewis S, Kirkman-Brown J, Coomarasamy A. The effect of sperm DNA fragmentation on miscarriage rates: a systematic review and meta-analysis. Hum Reprod. 2012 Oct;27(10):2908-17 ("Robinson 2012").

9 Johnson L, Petty CS, Porter JC, Neaves WB: Germ cell degeneration during postprophase of meiosis and serum concentrations of gonadotropins in young adult and older adult men. Biol Reprod. 1984; 31: 779-84.18;
Plastira K, Msaouel P, Angelopoulou R, Zanioti K, Plastiras A, Pothos A, Bolaris S, Paparisteidis N, Mantas D: The effects of age on DNA fragmentation, chromatin packaging and conventional semen parameters in spermatozoa of oligoasthenoteratozoospermic patients. J Assist Reprod Genet. 2007; 24: 437-43.
Siddighi 2007

10 Misell LM, Holochwost D, Boban D, Santi N, Shefi N, Hellerstein MK, Turek PJ: A stable isotope-mass spectrometric method for measuring human spermatogenesis kinetics in vivo. J Urol. 2006; 175: 242-6

11 Auger J, Eustache F, Andersen AG, Irvine DS, Jørgensen N, Skakkebaek NE, Suominen J, Toppari J, Vierula M, Jouannet P: Sperm morphological defects related to environment, lifestyle and medical history of 1001 male partners of pregnant women from four European cities. Hum Reprod. 2001; 16: 2710-7.

12 Armstrong JS, Rajasekaran M, Chamulitrat W, Gatti P, Hellstrom WJ, Sikka SC. Characterization of reactive oxygen species induced effects on human spermatozoa movement and energy metabolism. Free Radic. Biol. Med. 1999; 26: 869–80. 12 Kodama H, Yamaguchi R, Fukuda J, Kasai H, Tanaka T. Increased oxidative deoxyribonucleic acid damage in the spermatozoa of infertile male patients. Fertil. Steril. 1997; 68: 519–24. 13 Barroso G, Morshedi M, Oehninger S. Analysis of DNA fragmentation, plasma membrane translocation of phosphatidylserine and oxidative stress in human spermatozoa. Hum. Reprod. 2000; 15: 1338–44.

13 Mahfouz R, Sharma R, Thiyagarajan A, Kale V, Gupta S, Sabanegh E, Agarwal A. Semen characteristics and sperm DNA fragmentation in infertile men with low and high levels of seminal reactive oxygen species. Fertil Steril. 2010 Nov;94(6):2141-6.

14 Wong EW, Cheng CY. Impacts of environmental toxicants on male reproductive dysfunction. Trends Pharmacol Sci. 2011 May;32(5):290-9.

15 Esteves 2012.

16 Meseguer M, Martínez-Conejero JA, O'Connor JE, Pellicer A, Remohí J, Garrido N. The significance of sperm DNA oxidation in embryo development and reproductive outcome in an oocyte donation program: a new model to study a male infertility prognostic factor. Fertil Steril. 2008 May;89(5):1191-9.

17 Ross C, Morriss A, Khairy M, Khalaf Y, Braude P, Coomarasamy A, El-Toukhy T. A systematic review of the effect of oral antioxidants on male infertility. Reprod Biomed Online. 2010 Jun;20(6):711-23 ("Ross 2010"). Showell MG, Brown J, Yazdani A, Stankiewicz MT, Hart RJ. Antioxidants for male subfertility. Cochrane Database of Systematic Reviews (Online) 2011;11:CD007411 ("Showell 2011"); Robinson 2012.

18 Showell 2011.

19 Showell 2011.
20 Greco E, Romano S, Iacobelli M, Ferrero S, Baroni E, Minasi MG, Ubaldi F, Rienzi L, Tesarik J. ICSI in cases of sperm DNA damage: beneficial effect of oral antioxidant treatment. Hum Reprod. 2005 Sep;20(9):2590-4 ("Greco 2005b").
21 Ross C, Morriss A, Khairy M, Khalaf Y, Braude P, Coomarasamy A, El-Toukhy T. A systematic review of the effect of oral antioxidants on male infertility. Reprod Biomed Online. 2010 Jun;20(6):711-23.
22 Schmid TE, Eskenazi B, Marchetti F, Young S, Weldon RH, Baumgartner A, Anderson D, Wyrobek AJ. Micronutrients intake is associated with improved sperm DNA quality in older men. Fertil Steril. 2012 Nov;98(5):1130-7.e1
23 Mancini A, De Marinis L, Oradei A, Hallgass ME, Conte G, Pozza D, Littarru GP. Coenzyme Q10 concentrations in normal and pathological human seminal fluid. J Androl. 1994 Nov-Dec;15(6):591-4.
24 Lafuente R, González-Comadrán M, Solà I, López G, Brassesco M, Carreras R, Checa MA. Coenzyme Q10 and male infertility: a meta-analysis. J Assist Reprod Genet. 2013 Sep;30(9):1147-56; Nadjarzadeh A, Shidfar F, Amirjannati N, Vafa MR, Motevalian SA, Gohari MR, Nazeri Kakhki SA, Akhondi MM, Sadeghi MR. Effect of Coenzyme Q10 supplementation on antioxidant enzymes activity and oxidative stress of seminal plasma: a double-blind randomised clinical trial. Andrologia. 2013 Jan 7 ("Nadjarzadeh 2013").
Balercia 2009, Safarinejad 12.
25 Abad C, Amengual MJ, Gosálvez J, Coward K, Hannaoui N, Benet J, García-Peiró A, Prats J. Effects of oral antioxidant treatment upon the dynamics of human sperm DNA fragmentation and subpopulations of sperm with highly degraded DNA. Andrologia. 2013 Jun;45(3):211-6.
26 Nadjarzadeh 2013.
27 Safarinejad MR, Safarinejad S, Shafiei N, Safarinejad S. Effects of the reduced form of coenzyme Q10 (ubiquinol) on semen parameters in men with idiopathic infertility: a double-blind, placebo controlled, randomized study. J Urol. 2012 Aug;188(2):526-31.
28 Young SS, Eskenazi B, Marchetti FM, Block G, Wyrobek AJ. The association of folate, zinc and antioxidant intake with sperm aneuploidy in healthy non-smoking men. Hum Reprod. 2008 May;23(5):1014-22 ("Young 2008");

Mendiola J, Torres-Cantero AM, Vioque J, Moreno-Grau JM, Ten J, Roca M, Moreno-Grau S, Bernabeu R. A low intake of antioxidant nutrients is associated with poor semen quality in patients attending fertility clinics. Fertil Steril. 2010;11:1128–1133. Silver EW, Eskenazi B, Evenson DP, Block G, Young S, Wyrobek AJ. Effect of antioxidant intake on sperm chromatin stability in healthy nonsmoking men. J Androl. 2005 Jul-Aug;26(4):550-6.

29 Braga DP, Halpern G, Figueira Rde C, Setti AS, Iaconelli A Jr, Borges E Jr. Food intake and social habits in male patients and its relationship to intracytoplasmic sperm injection outcomes. Fertil Steril. 2012 Jan;97(1):53-9.

30 Young 2008.

31 Schmid TE, Eskenazi B, Marchetti F, Young S, Weldon RH, Baumgartner A, Anderson D, Wyrobek AJ. Micronutrients intake is associated with improved sperm DNA quality in older men. Fertil Steril. 2012 Nov;98(5):1130-7.e1.

32 Gupta NP, Kumar R (2002) Lycopene therapy in idiopathic male infertility—a preliminary report. Int Urol Nephrol 34(3):369– 372.

33 Huang XF, Li Y, Gu YH, Liu M, Xu Y, Yuan Y, Sun F, Zhang HQ, Shi HJ. The effects of Di-(2-ethylhexyl)-phthalate exposure on fertilization and embryonic development in vitro and testicular genomic mutation in vivo. PLoS One. 2012;7(11):e50465; Pant N, Pant A, Shukla M, Mathur N, Gupta Y, Saxena D. Environmental and experimental exposure of phthalate esters: the toxicological consequence on human sperm. Hum Exp Toxicol. 2011 Jun;30(6):507-14; Duty S. M., Singh N. P., Silva M. J., Barr D. B., Brock J. W., Ryan L., Herrick R. F., Christiani D. C., Hauser R. 2003b. The relationship between environmental exposures to phthalates and DNA damage in human sperm using the neutral comet assay. Environ. Health Perspect. 111, 1164–1169. ("In conclusion, this study represents the first human data to demonstrate that urinary MEP, at environmental levels, is associated with increased DNA damage in sperm.")

34 Mendiola J, Meeker JD, Jørgensen N, Andersson AM, Liu F, Calafat AM, Redmon JB, Drobnis EZ, Sparks AE, Wang C, Hauser R, Swan SH. Urinary concentrations of di(2-ethylhexyl) phthalate metabolites and serum reproductive hormones: pooled analysis of fertile and infertile men. J Androl. 2012 May-Jun;33(3):488-98. Meeker J. D., Calafat A.M., Hauser R. Urinary metabolites of di(2-ethylhexyl) phthalate are associated with decreased steroid hormone levels in adult men.. J Androl. 2009 May–Jun; 30(3): 287-297.

35 Ferguson KK, Loch-Caruso R, Meeker JD. Urinary phthalate metabolites in relation to biomarkers of inflammation and oxidative stress: NHANES 1999-2006. Environ Res. 2011 Jul;111(5):718-26.

36 Buck Louis G.M., Sundaram R., Sweeney A., Schisterman E.F., Kannan K. Bisphenol A, phthalates and couple fecundity, the life study. Fertil. Steril. 2013 Sep; 100(3): S1.

37 Meeker JD, Ehrlich S, Toth TL, Wright DL, Calafat AM, Trisini AT, Ye X, Hauser R. Semen quality and sperm DNA damage in relation to urinary bisphenol A among men from an infertility clinic. Reprod Toxicol. 2010 Dec;30(4):532-9.

38 Knez J, Kranvogl R, Breznik BP, Vončina E, Vlaisavljević V. Are urinary bisphenol A levels in men related to semen quality and embryo development after medically assisted reproduction? Fertil Steril. 2014 Jan;101(1):215-221.e5Li DK, Zhou Z, Miao M, He Y, Wang J, Ferber J, Herrinton LJ, Gao E, Yuan W. Urine bisphenol-A (BPA) level in relation to semen quality. Fertil Steril. 2011 Feb;95(2):625-30.e1-4.

39 Liu C, Duan W, Zhang L, Xu S, Li R, Chen C, He M, Lu Y, Wu H, Yu Z, Zhou Z. Bisphenol A exposure at an environmentally relevant dose induces meiotic abnormalities in adult male rats. Cell Tissue Res. 2014 Jan;355(1):223-32.

40 Wu HM, Lin-Tan DT, Wang ML, Huang HY, Lee CL, Wang HS, Soong YK, Lin JL. Lead level in seminal plasma may affect semen quality for men without occupational exposure to lead. Reprod Biol Endocrinol. 2012 Nov 8;10:91.
Telisman S, Colak B, Pizent A, Jurasović J, Cvitković P. Reproductive toxicity of low-level lead exposure in men. Environ Res. 2007 Oct;105(2):256-66.
Hernández-Ochoa I, García-Vargas G, López-Carrillo L, Rubio-Andrade M, Morán-Martínez J, Cebrián ME, Quintanilla-Vega B. Low lead environmental exposure alters semen quality and sperm chromatin condensation in northern Mexico. Reprod Toxicol. 2005 Jul-Aug; 20(2):221-8.

41 http://www.ewg.org/report/ewgs-water-filter-buying-guide

42 Arabi M, Heydarnejad MS. In vitro mercury exposure on spermatozoa from normospermic individuals. Pak J Biol Sci. 2007;10:2448–53.
Mohamed MK, Lee WI, Mottet NK, Burbacher TM. Laser light-scattering study of the toxic effects of methylmercury on sperm motility. J Androl. 1986;7:11–5.

Ernst E, Lauritsen JG. Effect of organic and inorganic mercury on human sperm motility. Pharmacol Toxicol. 1991;68:440–4.

43 Mocevic E, Specht IO, Marott JL, Giwercman A, Jönsson BA, Toft G, Lundh T, Bonde JP. Environmental mercury exposure, semen quality and reproductive hormones in Greenlandic Inuit and European men: a cross-sectional study. Asian J Androl. 2013 Jan;15(1):97-104

44 http://www.ewg.org/research/dirty-dozen-list-endocrine-disruptors

45 Sandhu RS, Wong TH, Kling CA, Chohan KR. In vitro effects of coital lubricants and synthetic and natural oils on sperm motility. Fertil Steril. 2014 Jan 23 [Epub ahead of print] ("Sandhu 2014"); Agarwal A, Deepinder F, Cocuzza M, Short RA, Evenson DP. Effect of vaginal lubricants on sperm motility and chromatin integrity: a prospective comparative study. Fertil Steril. 2008 Feb;89(2):375-9.

46 Sandhu 2014

47 Gaur DS, Talekar MS, Pathak VP. Alcohol intake and cigarette smoking: Impact of two major lifestyle factors on male fertility. Indian J Pathol Microbiol. 2010;11:35–40.
Muthusami KR, Chinnaswamy P. Effect of chronic alcoholism on male fertility hormones and semen quality. Fertil Steril. 2005;11:919–924

48 Klonoff-Cohen H, Lam-Kruglick P, Gonzalez C. Effects of maternal and paternal alcohol consumption on the success rates of in vitro fertilization and gamete intrafallopian transfer. Fertil Steril. 2003;79:330–9.

49 Braga DP, Halpern G, Figueira Rde C, Setti AS, Iaconelli A Jr, Borges E Jr. Food intake and social habits in male patients and its relationship to intracytoplasmic sperm injection outcomes. Fertil Steril. 2012 Jan;97(1):53-9.

50 Koch OR, Pani G, Borrello S et al. Oxidative stress and antioxidant defenses in ethanol-induced cell injury. Mol Aspects Med. 2004; 25: 191–8.

51 Agarwal A, Deepinder F, Sharma RK, Ranga G, Li J. Effect of cell phone usage on semen analysis in men attending infertility clinic: An observational study. Fertil Steril. 2008;11:124–128

52 Agarwal A, Desai NR, Makker K, Varghese A, Mouradi R, Sabanegh E, Sharma R. Effects of radiofrequency electromagnetic waves (RF-EMW) from cellular phones on human ejaculated semen: An in vitro pilot study. Fertil Steril. 2009;11:1318-1325.

53 Agarwal A, Singh A, Hamada A, Kesari K. Cell phones and male infertility: A review of recent innovations in technology and consequences. Int Braz J Urol. 2011;11:432–454.

54 Carlsen E, Andersson AM, Petersen JH, Skakkebaek NE. History of febrile illness and variation in semen quality. Hum. Reprod. 2003; 18: 2089–92.

55 Jung A, Leonhardt F, Schill W, Schuppe H. Influence of the type of undertrousers and physical activity on scrotal temperature. Hum Reprod. 2005;11:1022–1027

56 Tiemessen CH, Evers JL, Bots RS. Tight-fitting underwear and sperm quality. Lancet. 1996;11:1844–1845.

41457567R00182

Made in the USA
Middletown, DE
12 March 2017